Your Free Gift

Get Free Access to a 7-Day Meditation Program.

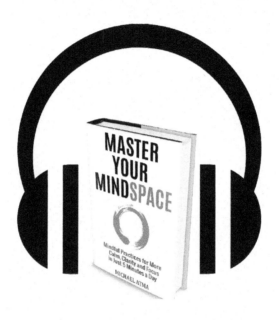

These seven guided meditations will give you greater calm, clarity and focus in just 5-minutes per day.

Or go to:

http://www.masteryourmindspace.com/meditationprogram

MASTER YOUR
MINDSPACE

Mindful Practices for More
Calm, Clarity and Focus
in Just 5 Minutes a Day

MICHAEL ATMA

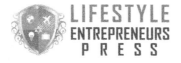
LIFESTYLE
ENTREPRENEURS
PRESS

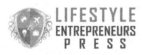 **Publisher: Jesse Krieger**

If you are interested in being published through Lifestyle Entrepreneurs Press, please email: Jesse@JesseKrieger.com

ACKNOWLEDGMENTS

I am deeply thankful to my teachers throughout the years, especially my meditation teachers, for their wisdom, guidance, and depth of being. Without them this book would never have been written.

I'd like to add a special thanks to everyone I have ever attended workshops, seminars, retreats and personal development programs with as your presence helped me to open the doors to parts of me that I would not have found on my own.

I'd also like to thank my mother and father for always believing in me and for giving me the ultimate gift – life. And last, but by no means least, I'd like to thank my wife Nadine, for her love, support, and unshakable trust in me and in what I do. It means the world to me.

TABLE OF CONTENTS

FOREWORD

"How are you doing"

'Good, just busy you know"

"Yeah, me too"

Does this conversation sound familiar? I hear it in some shape or form numerous times each day.

But busy with what?

It is all too easy to become busy without actually getting anything done. Or, perhaps worse, focusing exclusively on putting out daily fires and being reactive to other people's agendas at the expense of chasing our own most valuable goals and dreams.

In an increasingly connected world that is always on, it is more important now than perhaps ever before in the history of civilization to be the master of the space between our ears. To be the master of our mind, and to retire there for five minutes or so each day to zoom out and look at the big picture.

For without perspective and without clarity on our goals and objectives being busy does not equate to forward progress, but rather spinning our wheels in frustration; making a lot of noise but not really going anywhere.

There are a number of reasons why life seems to speed up and we are in a constant state of reactivity and "trying to keep up" with everything going on.

First and foremost is the advent of technology, and computing power in particular. While our brains and bodies have developed and evolved over the centuries and millennia, we have developed in a linear fashion. In the best of times, each generation making progress over the last in terms of life expectancy, quality of life and incremental improvement in the human condition.

Yet while humans have enjoyed incremental progress for all of history, the advent of computers and the rapid cycles of iteration and improvement to processing power has grown *exponentially*.

Let us say that over five generations, humans experience incremental improvement each generation, so starting at 1, by the end of five generations the quality of life has improved 1 + 1 + 1 + 1 + 1 = 5. In other words, five generations later an individual's quality of life is 5x that of their forebears.

But with technology, which is now so intertwined in our daily lives as to be nearly inseparable, computational power doubles with each generation according to Moore's Law – So now in five generations the processing power has grown 1 to 2, then 2 to 4, and 4 to 8, 8 to 16 and finally 16 to 32x the first generation. All other things the same, computational power has increased 32x over five generations of exponential growth while humans have increased 5x. That's quite a difference!

But it doesn't stop there, because computational power doubles in far less than a human lifetime. So the net effect is that in our lifetimes computers, technology and everything it touches will increase in power far beyond our own biology.

To me, this explains why time seems to speed up as I've grown older. Or, put another way, with an always-on news cycle and the sum total of the world's information accessible from a smart phone that's is nearly always by our side, the time between an important event happening and nearly everyone in the world knowing about it has decreased to nearly zero.

To be sure, there are numerous benefits to technology's advance; indeed it underpins many of the luxuries and amenities of modern society. And yet, one of the side effects is feeling a rush or pressure to "keep up" and find time to "get it all done".

Well here is the good news. Our mind is bound neither by our biology or the current state of technology, for our mind is capable of operating in "non-linear" terms!

In other words, while our biology improves incrementally, and technology scales exponentially, our mind sits above it all and can access memories of the past, tune into the present and envision a brighter future instantaneously.

You can prove this now by thinking back to a childhood memory. Got it? Now think about a goal that you're working towards in the future. And finally tune into the present moment and notice what is going on around you.

In a matter of seconds, you can traverse the span of your lifetime. You can contemplate ancient history, and speculate on what wonders the future may hold.

This is the non-linear power of the mind; our greatest asset to manifest what we want in life.

That is why it is of the utmost importance for you to understand the workings of your mind, and ultimately learn to Master Your Mindspace, which is what

Michael Atma teaches you over the course of this book.

Perhaps the greatest benefit to us as humans with a non-linear mind is that in a few short minutes we can divorce ourselves from whatever passion grips us in the moment and return to the quiet inner space where anything is possible.

From this place of infinite possibility, we can consciously turn our focus to the aspects of life that have real meaning and importance to us and reclaim our power over the unfolding of life, instead of feeling swept away in a current seemingly beyond our control.

In Master Your Mindspace, internationally recognized meditation teacher Michael Atma shares simple strategies to attain more calm, clarity and focus in just five minutes per day. This is accomplished through personal anecdotes and stories, as well as time-tested strategies and simple meditations that can put you back in control of your life and let you consciously guide it's unfolding.

I recommend that you read this book thoroughly and give yourself the gift of following his five-minute meditations. When you do, I believe you'll feel more grounded and clear with a renewed optimism and focus on that which truly matters to you.

So, sit back, relax and ease into your power with Master Your Mindspace!

To your success,

Jesse Krieger

Las Vegas, NV
#1 Best-Selling Author of Lifestyle Entrepreneur

INTRODUCTION

This book is the result of having the courage to dare to be different and live a non-traditional life. In my twenties I was at the peak of success as a corporate executive who traveled the world and was paid like a king only to have it all come crashing down when the company folded. What happened next took me on a 10-year world-wide adventure of self-discovery where I met remarkable teachers who helped me to free my mind and unleash my spirit.

But this book isn't about me – it's about You!

If you apply just one of the ideas or techniques in this book and put it into practice, it will change your life. I promise.

This book contains the essence of everything I've learned over the last 17 years of harnessing the power of the mind to live an extraordinary quality of life, get paid to do what I love and explore the things I am passionate about. Now I would like to share a blueprint for how you can do all of these things and so much more in just five minutes a day.

What exactly is mind-space? The best way I can answer that is to get you to think about a time when your mind was so peaceful and quiet and yet you were more alert than ever. This is what I call mind-space.

For some people this happens naturally while exercising, gardening, or doing anything at all that becomes meditative for them.

It's those moments when you stop thinking about what you are doing and suddenly find yourself being fully present in the moment.

When this happens a calmness and clarity arises within you. All thoughts of past or future dissolve leaving you feeling like you are in the flow of life and everything becomes simple, easy, and enjoyable.

In other words, it brings an instant relief to the never ending struggle that most of us experience trying to deal with the deluge of thoughts, feelings, and bodily sensations we experience from moment to moment.

Mind-space is also the gap between thoughts that happens when you are not thinking about anything in particular and suddenly an idea or answer to a problem pops into your head. Like when you are trying so hard to remember someone's name, who just happens to be standing in front of you, only to have it pop into your head the moment you stop thinking about it.

If you are clear in the mind you will be able to find solutions for every problem that arises in your mind.

But that's just a small part of mind-space. From the moment we wake up in the morning until we fall asleep at night, our minds are constantly working and moving from one thought and direction to another. This requires energy and if we never get a break from it then that's when mental, physical, and emotional suffering happens, which in turn affects our happiness and quality of life.

A mind that has no space for you to feel relaxed and in control of your life is a recipe for disaster. It's like being on a runaway train that you have no clue how to slow down or stop.

I learned a long time ago that the secret to a happy and productive life is to be the master of your mind and not its slave. I found that this begins with creating space in your head so that your mind and body can rest for a moment and re-charge. It makes sense then that the longer you can quiet your mind, the more recharged your body will be.

Mastering your mind-space is just the beginning. Once you know how to quiet your mind and give yourself space to be able to think clearly, breathe deeply and relax, then you will have the mental, emotional and physical resources to create anything you want in your life.

From being able to get and stay focused easier, through to doubling your productivity with less effort, there's no end to the life-transforming benefits that come from achieving a little bit of mind-space each day.

Up until I started mastering my mind-space I was plagued by stress, anxiety and feeling like my life had no purpose or meaning. I turned to alcohol as a coping mechanism and found myself wandering from one job to the next, and one relationship to the next, looking to find happiness, love, and fulfillment. But instead all I found was dissatisfaction and disillusion.

Then, one day in my late twenties, I attended a four week self-improvement program called 'Mind Powers'. What happened for me at that event was so profound that it was to change the course of my life forever. This introduced me to the power of the mind and just how much control we don't have over it when our past conditioning causes us to make decisions and take actions that limit the amount of happiness, health, wealth, and freedom we can enjoy.

True freedom in life comes when we are no longer a slave to a mind that causes us to think and behave in crazy ways. As someone who wants to take charge of their life you must first learn how your mind works and what impact the way you think and behave influences your results. This will help you to get to know your mind and why your life is the way it is, and what you can do to change it.

In the process of exploring what it means to master your mind-space, I will share some stories from my own journey as both a student and a teacher, and present the learning lessons gained from these experiences.

Then I will show you the exact strategies and techniques that accelerated my personal and professional success, as well as helped me to find a deep place of rest within me that I can go to anytime and anywhere I want. Most of them will literally only take you five minutes to learn and apply and offer an experience of what they can do for you.

These are the same tools that helped to unlock my creativity and helped me to write and publish a book that sold over 8,000 copies, become an international public speaker, and now become a successful entrepreneur with three companies that are helping thousands of people world-wide to lead a better quality of life.

It is my deepest desire that this book inspires you to make changes to your life and to let go of those things that are holding you back from living, laughing, and loving deeply. As you go through it do not be surprised if you have a multitude of 'aha' moments as well as a renewed feeling of vitality to help you get more done in less time and with less effort.

Towards the end of the book I've included some simple yet powerful meditation techniques that will be useful for both beginners and experienced meditation enthusiasts to switch your mind off for a few moments and enjoy the multitude of benefits that come from being deeply relaxed.

The real power of this book though is to help you to have a deeper relationship within yourself and to create your life from a space of having a clear mind, a peaceful life, and being free to explore those things you are most passionate about.

Once the book ends, then the real journey begins. There is a rapidly growing community of Mindspace Masters that are using these ideas and techniques to change their lives and live their dreams.

I would love for you to join us so that we can connect with as many like-minded people as possible to learn and grow from each other in ways that would not be possible if we tried to figure it all out on our own.

For now, let's get started on your journey to Master Your Mindspace. If along the way you need to clarify anything or simply want to share an experience you had from using any of the techniques, then you can contact me at michael@michaelatma.com

I hope this book gives you the inspiration to live a life you love and enjoy, and gives you all the tools you need to do so.

MIND OVER MATTER

He who knows others is wise;
He who knows himself is enlightened
.- The Way of Lao-tzu

We all have dreams about how we want our life to be. For some it's to simply enjoy a happy, healthy and peaceful life, while for others it's to find and live that special gift that we believe deep down in our souls that we all have, so that we can make a difference, and make the world a better place.

Yet, for many of us, those dreams have become buried under the frustrations and demands of daily life to the point where we barely remember they are there, let alone strive to achieve them. Many have lost the spark inside that dreams keep alight – and with it, so has the power to change their lives.

My life's journey has been to restore the spark and awaken the dreams to make it a part of my everyday life, and to get each of us to enjoy a quality of life that we desire and deserve. This began as a quest to get to get to know myself better and led me down a path of awakening a silent power that lies sleeping in us all. This power is the unlimited power of a mind that is calm, clear and has controlled focus. Then, you can use your mind like a laser beam to cut through anything that might be stopping you from getting what you want.

Imagine what it would be like to wake-up each day and be passionate, happy, and grateful, instead of being tired, unmotivated, and frustrated. My obsession with having a life of passion and purpose began with some simple questions. "How can I take control of my life? What can I do today to be happier, healthier, and more empowered? How can I harness the power of my mind, and then share that with others in a meaningful and enjoyable way?"

Somewhere along the way I developed the belief that I could do anything I set my mind to. That wasn't something I was born with, but it appeared in my mind when I was ready for it. You see, I truly believe that each of us has hidden talents, gifts, and dreams that are unique for us, that when unleashed gives the opportunity to experience life to the fullest.

Everything you need to create the life you desire and deserve is available to you right now. It's waiting patiently inside you for the right time to appear. It's just that we get pre-occupied with things that we 'think' are important but after a while realize that they were the reason that we ended up staying stuck in a rut.

Wanting something badly will not make it happen. It will only happen when you change your thinking.

Just think back to the jobs that you left, or the relationships that ended, or the friends you used to have that you no longer see. What happened to these things? You changed how you thought about those things - that's what happened.

Whenever you change and open up to new ways of thinking and behaving you can bank on the fact that new opportunities are already on their way. Why? Because that's the way life works.

The Inner Child

From childhood, we learn most of what we know through repetition. Everything you believe you can or can't be has come about from what you were told was true about you and the experiences you had that reinforced your beliefs. That's why if you were told often enough that you weren't good enough, smart enough, strong enough, or worthy enough to follow your dreams, then what chance did you have of letting your inner light shine through?

In fact, by the time we are seven years old, most of our dreams have been forgotten because of the need to conform to 'rules'. Rules are not a bad thing to have in life. Certain boundaries are necessary in our world otherwise there would be more chaos than there is already.

They do, however, have a huge impact on our subconscious-mind and the beliefs that we live by. If you grow up believing that you have to 'do as you are told', then you will most likely have difficulty expressing yourself in a creative or empowered way.

If what you have to say, do, or share is not valued by others in the formative years of your life, how can you ever expect that to be any different as an adult? This is why many people don't feel confident to express themselves openly and honestly. The downside of this is that you cheat yourself out of living fully. Here's a good question to ask yourself, "What rules do I live by, my own, or the ones I have borrowed from others?"

A simple way to tell if you are happy with what you do in your everyday life is if you enjoy your work, relationships, friends and family, then you are living by your rules. If you don't then someone else's rules are in charge.

Most people think they work in jobs they don't like because they have to pay the mortgage or feed their family, but this is not true. It is your inner beliefs about who you are and what you can do that influences the choices you make in life.

You have to learn the rules of the game. Only then can you know which ones to break to play bigger and better than anyone else.

This is why some people seem to get what they want, while others don't. It's how good they get at identifying rules that hold them back and then breaking the pattern in their life.

In my seminars one of the most common things I find is that most people don't know what they want. This is why they put up with less than what they could have, be, or do. When you have anything in your life that you don't enjoy it is because you haven't yet discovered what you do want.

When I was in my twenties I started looking for more meaning in my life. After traveling the world for three years and meeting the most extraordinary people who showed me things about myself that I probably wouldn't have learned in seventy years of conventional living, I knew there was no turning back.

I got to see just how many limiting rules I had bought into that were controlling the level of happiness, health, love, prosperity, and freedom I could have in my life.

With great gusto I began to break down the walls holding these rules together and that's when everything began to change almost faster than I could keep up with.

HERE'S HOW TO SPEND THE NEXT 5 MINUTES

Write down an area of your life you are not happy with. Then see if you can identify a limiting rule that you are hanging on to and write it down. Next, take that piece of paper and burn it (safely of course). As it is burning say out loud, "I am so happy to be letting go of a part of me I no longer need."

Now, you are energetically free from this part of your past and it's time to move forward a little lighter and a whole heap brighter. This exercise is an invigorating healing tool that will take five minutes or less of your day.

Taking Charge of the Mind

I believe that we all have the potential to live a creative, inspired, rewarding, and absolutely joyful life. The first key in attaining this goal is to be the master of your mind, rather than its slave. In other words, your mind can either work for, or against you. It all depends upon how you focus it.

To focus on what's wrong with your life, what you can't do and how tough things are is to be a victim. To focus on what's right with your life, what you can do and how grateful you are is the path of victory.

To master your mind is to be disciplined. An undisciplined mind leads to:

29

- Confusion and frustration

- Excess stress and anxiety

- Lack of focus

- Self doubt and fear

- Poor work performance

- Inefficient time management

- Making rash decisions

- Making excuses

- Bad habits

- Addictions

- Low or no motivation

- Low energy levels

While, on the other hand, a disciplined mind develops:

- Improved concentration
- Clarity
- Inspiration
- Decisiveness
- Improved work performance
- Efficient time management
- Higher productivity
- More resistance to stress and pressure
- Effective habits
- High energy levels

While many people consider discipline to be hard work I have found it quite the opposite. At first, if you are not a highly motivated person, you may need to put a little effort into creating habits that benefit you. That's all discipline is really—a habit.

Just by taking five minutes a day to do something different that is going to help you to clear your mind or be more focused, is a nice micro-habit to get you started. It's the consistent small steps over time that matters when it comes to growth and change.

HERE'S HOW TO SPEND THE NEXT 5 MINUTES

Learning how to develop and concentrate your thoughts so that they become more powerful is one of the biggest investments you can make with your time and energy. For this exercise, just close your eyes and count to ten and then back down to one again. Repeat this for five minutes. When your mind wanders which it will, come back to counting. That's it. Everything you need to start taking control of your mind is in this simple mindfulness technique.

Center Yourself

We are all born with a center, but many don't even know it exists. We can live without knowing our center, but we can't be without it. If you do not have a connection to your center, you will feel out of balance with both your inner reality and your outer world.

Your center is the place inside you that feels like home. In martial arts it is called the "center-point", or "Hara", which is said to reside in the lower belly region of the body, and when translated means 'ocean of energy'.

Regardless of what it is called, it is a space within me that I have come to know very well. At any time of the day or night I can bring my awareness to my center and experience instantaneous calm and clarity. In fact as I write about it now it washes over my mind and body in waves making me feel deeply relaxed and at peace.

There is nothing mystical about this space at all. It lives within all of us. We just need to remember that it is there and then consciously connect to it. More than anything, connecting to your center brings you fully into the present moment. It is the simplest way to get out of your head, into your body, and be-here-now. All it takes is awareness.

Once you master this knack, then your life will take on a whole new meaning. If you look around you at all the people whose lives appear to be empty and meaningless to them, or they are caught up in suffering and struggle, you will find that they are all living without connecting to their center.

They are allowing thoughts, feelings, events, and circumstances to throw them around like washing in a spin drier without any hope of having a place to rest in and re-charge their mind and bodies. Even a tornado has a center that is quiet and peaceful. No matter how strong or destructive the winds are on the outside of it, the center remains untouched.

Our center works just the same. On the outside our lives can be driving us crazy mentally, physically and emotionally, but deep inside us we have a center that never gets touched by these things. I'm sure you have experienced this for yourself at some point in your life but the real secret to tapping into its power is to connect with it consciously whenever you want.

To connect with your center on a regular basis and be able to enjoy knowing it as a part of who you are, is to have a deep connection with your inner being. This provides you with an energetic anchor to a more stable foundation of life that no amount of money, power, people, or external things can ever provide.

It is by far one of the biggest kept secrets to getting rid of fear, anxiety and anguish from your life. Imagine that, just by being centered you can instantly be free from the distractions of the mind and the world that cause us to suffer.

It may sound too good to be true, but the truth is that the greatest gifts that life has to offer come from the simplest of things. Centering yourself is one of them – it is so easy to do, we just have to remember that we have one and then the craziness of the moment drops away like magic.

Don't just take my word for it though – try it for yourself.

HERE'S HOW TO SPEND THE NEXT 5 MINUTES

Close your eyes and take a few moments to relax. Once you are settled, scan your body with your awareness, and ask it to show you where your center is located. Then, when you become aware of where your center point is located in your body – place your hands there.

As you gently place your hands over the part of your body that feels like your center point just keep your awareness on the connection between your hands and center. You may even feel some heat in your hands or body at this stage. If you have found your center then you may also notice that your mind is crystal clear and alert, and that you feel deeply rooted in your body.

For the first few times you practice connecting with your center it may help to use your hands so that you can more easily connect to it with your mind. After a while though, make the connection without your hands and you should notice that it will happen easier and quicker. Eventually you will be able to close your eyes and make the connection instantly. Then you can do it anywhere and anytime you want to.

California Dreaming

Do you believe that dreams can come true? Last year, I participated in a five-day 'success seminar' in California. Hundreds of people attended from all over the world to either know, or grow their heart's desire. Some of us knew what our dreams were. Others had no idea.

Each day we gathered together in small groups to share our knowledge, skills, and ideas. The purpose of this was to develop the tools of supporting and being supported, using teamwork to make the dream work.

Jill was a single mum who joined one of my teams. Her dream was to sing and record children's songs. The challenge for us was that Jill had no singing experience and was too nervous and embarrassed to perform in front of other people.

Our group had no idea what Jill's voice sounded like, so our first priority was to find a way to encourage her to sing for us.

We came up with a plan that involved creating a space where Jill felt comfortable enough to let go of her inhibitions and sing. We hired a soundproof music booth and left Jill alone in there with some of her favorite songs, saying that we would be back in one hour.

What Jill did not know was that we would be able to hear her from a room that was set up to monitor her progress. It worked magnificently.

We discovered that Jill had a beautiful voice so then we knew that we could help her realize her dream.

Putting our heads together we found some nursery rhymes that Jill liked and within six months she had recorded her first children's album. That album was so successful that Jill immediately went to work recording a second one.

These days, Jill writes her own lyrics, runs her own production company, gets paid for what she loves to do, and wakes up each day thankful to be alive.

Finding your dream can sometimes be just as challenging as living it. After spending your entire life living out other people's dreams, it's no wonder that finding your own can be confusing.

Never fear though, because your dreams will be awakened at exactly the right time for you. In the meantime, learning to enjoy the life you already have is a big step in the right direction.

HERE'S HOW TO SPEND THE NEXT 5 MINUTES

Do something that you wouldn't normally do that is just for you. Just imagine for a moment that you are completely free to be anything you want to be and that it's okay to say yes to yourself... just for five minutes. Make sure it's something that you'll enjoy doing and which is fun for you. By doing this you are giving yourself permission to shine.

If In Doubt - DO IT!

What is it that you can do to create a better life for yourself? Right now, in this moment, is there something you have been putting off doing that could benefit you or others? Is there a phone call you could make, a letter you could write, or action you could take to demonstrate your willingness to let go of the past and get on with creating a bigger, brighter, and more powerful future?

Never doubt for a moment that you have the power to change your life in an instant. I have found that lingering in the background and waiting for life to change around me is a fool's errand.

This shows a lack of willingness to take responsibility for the way my life *is*. Every day, I allocate time and energy towards turning my dreams into reality, no matter how big or small they might be.

No matter what desires you have such as:

- Financial independence
- More intimate relationships
- Increased self-confidence
- A bigger house
- More time
- Improved health and fitness
- Four holidays a year
- Singing lessons
- A longer life
- To sack your boss

Nothing is impossible to achieve - *if you know how.*

Knowledge is easily attainable. There are libraries filled with all kinds of information on 'how to' do almost anything, not to mention the internet. If that doesn't work, then there are people all over the world who are ready, willing, and able to share their success secrets with you, sometimes for a price, sometimes for free.

Regardless of what you want to achieve in your life, somewhere near you there is someone or something that can get you started and help you through any turbulent times. All you have to do is look or ask for help when you need it. Be careful of stubborn or prideful attitudes because they can turn a short journey into an epic.

Kicking the Habit

After many years of walking along a pathway of self-discovery, I have come to realize that there is more of everything. If you want more happiness, then you can have it. If you want more financial freedom, then you can have it. If you want better health, then you can have it. Even if you want more misery or stress, then you can have that also.

It all depends where you choose to focus your attention. I have seen many people open the doors to joyful living, only to watch them fight tooth and nail to prove to themselves that they are not worthy to be happy.

It may sound absurd, but the absurdity is that it is true. It is a fact that people are creatures of habit. Some habits allow growth, flow, pleasure, and balance, while other habits keep us stuck on the treadmill of pain.

Being able to recognize habits that sabotage your ability to live fully and freely is a major step forward in becoming more successful than you already are. Habits are neither good nor bad of their own accord. They are either conscious (known) or subconscious (unknown).

The more aware you become of sabotaging habits, the less influence they have over the quality of your life. These habits weave their way into your life like an unseen intruder in the night.

Just as you would turn on the light to confront the uninvited guest in your house, so too must you turn on the light of your conscious mind to release the negative influence of subconscious habits.

In My Opinion

For the first twenty five years of my life most of the opinions I had about myself were based upon the world around me and what I had achieved.

I had no idea that my perceptions of who I believed I was were rigid and superficial. Then my girlfriend at the time came home one evening and asked me to do a four-week personal growth course with her.

I responded with a typically arrogant male attitude of, "I don't need to develop anything. I am quite happy the way I am", feeling secure within myself that nothing short of an earthquake would sway me.

My girlfriend replied with, "I want us to do this course together to help our relationship". Now she had my full attention. I had no idea that our relationship needed "help". Where had I been hiding all of this time?

Over the next four weeks many scary and exciting experiences filled my life. My opinions about myself, other people, and life in general were no longer as concrete as they used to be. My confident, organized, and usually flamboyant personality felt like it had been thrown into a gigantic washing machine.

Sometimes, I felt like I was out of control and desperately wished I could find somewhere to hide until my life returned to 'normal'. However, some part of me knew that no matter where I went, who I was with, or what I did, I would not be able to escape the changes that were happening because they were coming from inside me.

As time went by I came to understand that I was letting go of old beliefs and ideas about myself at a deep subconscious level. By this, I mean that somehow my conditioned beliefs about myself were being released without me consciously doing anything and a more authentic part of me was surfacing to be lived.

Pretty soon, I noticed that many of my habits had changed. I began to eat different foods, as if I had been doing it all my life. I started meeting new people and going places and doing things that I would never have dreamed of before. It was as if suddenly I had a whole new life and I felt lighter, freer, and happier than I could remember.

The challenge is that your ego gets attached to what it knows, whether it's good for you or not. It's a bit like a child who needs a safety blanket to go to sleep at night. The only reason the blanket is needed is because the child is afraid and the blanket helps it to calm down.

This is the same with many of your beliefs. Without them you can become lost and frightened. Even if your life is full of drama or negative experiences, the truth is that without them, your mind that is conditioned to believe in these things as acceptable in your life would most likely freak out if it didn't have them.

So you might go on smoking cigarettes, drinking alcohol, worrying about the future and feeling guilty about the past, or living in lack, and being miserable, all because your conditioned mind is addicted to these things.

Before you get up in arms about this statement just consider the possibility that the only rational reason you might sabotage your health, prosperity, peace of mind or happiness is because some part of you wants to. The fact that you have not been aware of it until now is irrelevant.

You can never change these patterns unless you can accept this statement. Self-sabotaging belief systems float around in your subconscious like mini thought forms seeking to undermine everything your conscious mind thinks it wants.

No one in their right mind would ever put smoke into their lungs, yet something inside 30% of adult males and females creates this behavior. Isn't it strange that very few people ever look closely at why they say, think or do some of the crazy things they do? What's even stranger is that many people that I come across say they don't care.

Of course they don't care while their body appears to be okay. But watch what happens when the body starts to show signs of deteriorating. Everything from panic and anxiety, to disbelief and depression sets in. In many cases, these life-threatening illnesses could have been easily prevented through making better life choices.

Almost everything that happens to you is in some way caused by you. If this is true, then surely it makes sense that you have the power to make choices that bring you more positive outcomes.

Self-sabotaging belief systems will always be a part of your life until you no longer need them. The day you no longer need them is the day you start being 100% responsible for your life and stop being a victim. Then their power to control your destiny fades away.

HERE'S HOW TO SPEND THE NEXT 5 MINUTES

Make a decision right now to give up one thing in your life that is sabotaging your happiness, health, relationships, or finances. Write down the old behavior on a piece of paper and then go burn it. As it burns say out loud, *"I am so happy to be letting go of a part of me that no longer serves me."*

Jewel of the Smile

Throughout this journey I will continue to share my insights in a way that will assist in unleashing the awesome potential that exists within you to change your life for the better.

Within every one of us lie magnificent jewels waiting to be discovered. These jewels vary from person to person and can be any shape or size, yet they will always dazzle you with their brilliance once they are uncovered.

You may be a gifted musician, healer, teacher, artist, sculptor, poet, writer, dancer, or have any number of talents and skills waiting to be expressed.

Never compare your special gifts or talents with those of others. Your contribution to life matters just as much as anyone else's. The precious gem that lives within your heart and soul only needs a little encouragement to flow naturally and powerfully into the world.

You will know when this happens because you will always have a smile on your face and your heart and mind will be at peace.

Be patient with yourself as your inner awakening unfolds. It may take time to come to full fruition but the wait will certainly be worthwhile. In the meantime, start doing things that you have always wanted to do and somehow never got around to. You may be pleasantly surprised at the results you achieve.

HERE'S HOW TO SPEND THE NEXT 5 MINUTES

Decide on a new hobby that you'd like to take up. It may be something that you started in the past but it got pushed aside as life got in the way, or it may be something you've always wanted to do but never got around to doing it.

Then spend the next five minutes checking out who, where, what, or how you can get started and book a time and date to do it.

IMAGINE YOUR SELF

The Blending of Two Worlds

There is no limit to the amount of happiness, calmness, health, wealth, success, or love that you can have. The only limits that exist are the ones that are created through inflexible habits and beliefs.

You may not always be aware of the hidden influences that lessen the quality of your life, yet, like the unseen wind, they exist and have power.

The evidence of this can be found in the circumstances you find yourself in and what beliefs you have regarding your self-image. Whenever you suffer, for any reason at all, you can be sure that unseen forces are at work undermining the foundation of your self-image.

This unseen force belongs to your inner critic. It only exists to remind you that you still judge your worthiness to live in joy.

Improving your self-image takes more than exercising your body, buying a bigger house, or being polite to everyone. It also requires opening up to your inner self so that you can discover the strength, beauty, and wealth of love that exists both within and around you.

You can achieve this regardless of how much money you have or don't have, the state of your health, or the circumstances that you have created. Why waste time going from one place to another, one job to the next, or one relationship to another, when what you are really searching for has been right under your very nose all along?

While your ego continues to struggle to modify your outer life in an attempt to be fulfilled, you will only know a superficial existence. Your inner world is vast and expansive, while your outer world remains limited and superficial.

As long as your happiness or misery is influenced by what goes on outside of you, you are not in charge of your life. Just like a puppet has its body controlled by strings in the hands of a puppeteer, you too can have your 'strings' pulled by people or events around you as long as you give away your power to them to control you.

What about all those times you were convinced that you would be happy when you found the right job, the right partner, when your debts were paid, or when some future-based event was to happen? When those things did happen, or if they never happened at all, only then did you realize that you still experienced the same emptiness and frustration.

The moment you fulfill any desire you will feel this emptiness and frustration. It is desire that fuels your actions, not the goal. Goals are only intended to be bridges to build your passion for life, they are never meant to be attained.

This is why your goals are always changing. You can never be wholly satisfied with what you have, until you have either saturated your desires or let them go. For the moment, consider that...

Your mind doesn't know the difference
between what you do want or don't want.
It only knows what you focus on.

Many people focus on what they don't have, what they 'can't' do, and their limitations. As a result, they end up experiencing more of these.

Power-Full Living

As I grew up I believed that power came from physical effort. I spent many years studying martial arts, training at the gym and developing physical prowess. It wasn't until I began to see how limited my beliefs were that I began to explore the multifaceted nature of power and the impact it has in shaping our future.

I discovered that there are two main types of power that shape the way our lives look.

The first is conscious power. This means that you are in charge of your life, have awareness of the consequence of your actions and understand that life is created from the inside-out.

The second is unconscious power. This means that you are a victim of circumstances, have no idea as to the consequence of your actions, and believe that life is created from the outside-in.

Here are some powers of pleasure and pain that influence the quality of your life:

PLEASURE	PAIN
The power of love	The power of anger

The power of choice	The power of suffering
The power of action	The power of greed
The power of joy	The power of rejection
The power of energy	The power of misery
The power of success	The power of failure
The power of beauty	The power of control
The power of passion	The power of judgment
The power of pleasure	The power of guilt

For the next seven days, at the end of each day write down whatever experiences or feelings you remember having during the day and note alongside them what powers you have used.

For example, if you had an argument with a loved one, then some of the powers you explored could be pain, judgment, guilt, misery, criticism, compliance, and deception. Then if you both made-up, the powers you used could look like love, joy, happiness, forgiveness, compassion, and humility.

Note which powers appear to be happening most frequently and you will start to understand where you are focusing your energy and why your life is the way it is.

There are no accidents when it comes to what you create in your life. There is only action and reaction. In other words, what you put out from you in the energy of your thoughts, words, and actions is what you get back.

Once you identify where you are focusing on powers that reinforce negativity, lack, unhappiness, or misery, then you will have the power to transform any area of your life in an instant!

By choosing to use powers that benefit you in a constructive way you can ensure that you are giving yourself the best opportunity to release painful patterns of behavior and embrace pleasurable ones.

HERE'S HOW TO SPEND THE NEXT 5 MINUTES

Write down what powers are influencing your life right now. Are they in alignment with what you want to achieve for yourself? If not, spend five minutes deciding which power you most need to focus on in order to move forward with your life's goals. Know that there is nothing that can stop you from becoming this power as long as you never stop claiming more of it for yourself.

Which View Do You Prefer?

Imagine for a moment that you are standing inside a room and this room has four walls, and each wall has a small, single window in it. You are standing looking out of the east window and you can see a river that winds its way down from a majestic mountain range.

The top of the mountains are lightly covered with powdery snow, the sky is a dazzling blue, and a few gentle white clouds can be seen lazily drifting overhead.

The other three windows each have a person standing in front of them, looking out at something completely different to you. You are not able to see what the others are looking at because the windows are small and their bodies are blocking any possible view.

This is precisely how life works. All too often we are so caught up in our perspective that either we can't be bothered, or don't take the time to consider what other views are available to be enjoyed.

What's Your Allowance Level?

The next time you feel yourself getting angry with someone just stop for a moment and put yourself in their shoes.

- What has their day been like?
- How are they feeling?
- What is life like for them at the moment?
- You don't have to understand - just allow.

Be genuinely considerate towards their needs and your anger will turn into compassion. Allow that their view of life at the moment is right for them. This will teach you a profound lesson about yourself.

For most of us, our window to the world is our eyes. Even though everyone's eyes may see the same thing, our minds interpret them differently. The images outside never change, only the interpretations of them are different. Get the picture?

Interpretation (judgment) is what creates differences of opinion, conflicts, and challenges in your life. If everyone were to look at life through the same window and have the same interpretations of what they were looking at, then harmony and happiness would happen naturally.

Consider the possibility that your point of view is right for you and someone else's point of view is right for them and you will discover the tremendous healing power of *compassion.*

Opening to Self Trust

Trust is a big deal for many people. It is also something that is somewhat misunderstood. Some equate trust to honesty, but that is just the tip of the iceberg. It goes much deeper than that.

Consider for a moment that self trust means, "I am okay - no matter what."

This means that you become more accepting of the situations that you create and learn to flow with what is happening right now.

How could you possibly hope to trust another human being if you have not yet embraced those parts of you that you consider unpleasant or painful?

On a recent overseas tour, I learned the meaning of self-trust. Having been involved in running personal development seminars and workshops for several years, I decided to leave it all behind for a while and see what else the world had to offer.

My first stop was Hawaii. Four 'sun' soaked days later, a "chance" encounter with a local led me to a remote cove, where dolphins and whales played in abundance, and very few people gathered.

I felt like I was dreaming. As I gazed upon the beauty, tranquility and solitude of the mountains, trees, water, sand, and marine life, a deep contentment arose within my soul.

Suddenly, a pod of dolphins leapt out of the water less than fifty feet away from where I was standing. Like a child at an amusement park, I dropped my things, grabbed a snorkel, goggles, and flippers, and dove into the inviting blue ocean. As soon as my head went underwater I heard the dolphins "clicking" to each other.

After a few minutes, my entire body began to tingle with excitement as a pod of one hundred dolphins glided a few feet beneath me. They showed me how willing they were to play by rolling on their backs and waving; swimming in circles; jumping over me, and serenading me with a symphony of sounds from their sonar.

This experience was so profound that I stayed in Hawaii for six months. Some days at the cove there were strong currents, stormy skies, choppy seas, huge swells, and all kinds of conditions to endure, but what never ceased to amaze me was how unimportant these things were while I swam with my dolphin friends.

Many great things happened during this time. I had never been a strong swimmer in the past but now I could easily swim for hours at a time and come out feeling more energized and alive than when I went in. The dolphins were also teaching me that if you flow with the current of life, then much adventure will come your way.

From the first day that I decided to follow my heart without hesitation, and trust that I had the necessary courage, commitment and capacity to discover a life of joy and fulfillment, my vision of life soared to new levels.

Since that time, my dreams have changed. Now, I stand on the threshold of a new era and with deep gratitude in my heart for all of the experiences that have led me here, I embrace my destiny wholeheartedly by giving birth to the dreams that are alive within me now.

HERE'S HOW TO SPEND THE NEXT 5 MINUTES

Where in your life can you allow more trust? One of the fastest ways to have more trust in your life is to start giving more trust to others. Even letting someone do something for you that you would rather keep control of, demonstrates trust.

Write down where you have the least amount of trust and decide on an action you can take to demonstrate to yourself that you are willing to open to deeper levels of trust.

Never have an expectation of what the outcome is going to be when you give your trust. Instead, learn to flow with whatever happens and find a way to be at peace with it. Then, you will find true freedom in relationships and life.

The Perfect Balance

What an incredible gift it is to be alive in this day and age. We have more comfort, food, connectivity, and opportunities than ever before. No other generation has had such abundance at their disposal. Yet unhappiness is ripe throughout the world.

Things like stress, road rage, drug addiction, domestic violence, child abuse, unemployment, and disappearing family and social values, all indicate that something is out of balance.

If everything on the outside is more abundant, then the answer to our lack can only come from within. Unless we are able to give to ourselves what we need from the inside, then how can we possibly enjoy what we have on the outside?

I have come across many people searching to find meaning and value in their lives through the medium of the world around them. The common thread is a mixture of hope and futility. Although it can be a lot of fun exploring the outer world, it can also be quite empty on the inside.

The beauty of getting to know yourself from the inside-out is that balance occurs naturally, it doesn't need to be found. There can never be permanent harmony in your life until you are at peace with your entire existence. To be at peace with your existence, you must go within and rediscover your childlike innocence and enthusiasm for life.

Once you uncover these qualities that are buried beneath a lifetime of conditioning and compromise, you will no longer need to find anything because your life will be complete.

This does not mean that you will not get to travel, make love, have a family or do any of the things you enjoy doing. It means that you will discover even more things to enjoy and those things you already love will be even more fulfilling.

At first, going within and getting to know yourself better can be a little uncomfortable because your ego has to let go of being in control of what it knows and feels comfortable with. It can sometimes be a little like letting a bucking bronco out of its corral, but as time passes your ego calms down and the ride gets smoother.

As you look more deeply into yourself with awareness many of those qualities that you value the most such as calmness, confidence, trust and happiness just to name a few, automatically blossom within you.

Becoming more aware, or mindful, as it is called these days, of what's happening for you from moment to moment is the mechanism that enables you to look beyond your natural reactive behavior to external triggers such as stress or conflict and gives you space to gain insights at a different level of understanding.

When this happens, then you have the opportunity for new perceptions to arise that can help you to drop any needless suffering you may have been experiencing and instead find peace and relief.

Getting to know yourself at a deeper level of awareness happens naturally when you stop looking for answers from anyone else but you.

Whether you are breathing or walking, angry or sad, embrace it with mindfulness and watch as you transform suffering to relief.

A Lesson in Mindfulness

Mindfulness is simply being aware of here and now. It can be done while breathing, sitting, eating, driving or any time at all. One of the things that's not so well known about mindfulness though is that it also applies to feelings, thoughts, and bodily sensations.

To be mindful of one's feelings, especially the ones that can cause suffering like anger, rage, grief, depression, and many more like them is to be able to embrace them tenderly and look more deeply into the emotion. When you do this, then this brings a new awareness or understanding of it, which helps heal any misconceptions you may have been holding onto that were causing you to suffer.

This new understanding that arises from being mindful of any negative thoughts or feelings allows the opportunity for a profound transformation to take place for you in real-time.

As you stay aware of your thoughts or feelings and gently accept them with awareness and you start to have a new understanding of what is causing them, then compassion arises and with it comes relief and less suffering.

Mindfulness is a powerful tool to help create space in your life. The more space you have to look more deeply into your experience of the moment, the more compassion and peace you will find. It's only when we try to avoid our thoughts and feelings, or pretend that they don't exist that we end up becoming overwhelmed with the clutter of our own doing.

Mindfulness is how you will find a deeper happiness, health, and peace in your life than you ever dreamed possible. Try it for yourself right now and see how it works for you.

HERE'S HOW TO SPEND THE NEXT 5 MINUTES

Gently close your eyes and for the next minute or so, simply watch your thoughts come and go as if they are fluffy white clouds floating by in the sky. All you're doing is noticing your thoughts.

No matter what thought comes up, simply allow it to be okay and then let it go. If you find yourself getting hooked into any particular thought, then remind yourself that you are simply sitting and observing your thoughts and there is nothing to do and nowhere to go.

Then, gently open your eyes for a moment, stretch your body and then settle back down into your chair and close your eyes. For the next few minutes, simply be aware of your body. Notice where your body touches the chair, or whatever you are sitting on. Feel that connection. Then be aware of any sensations you may be feeling such as tightness, discomfort, or even if you are feeling hot or cold anywhere. Allow yourself to simply observe these sensations one at a time and don't try to change or get rid of them – just let them be. This is what it feels like to put mindfulness into motion and be-here-now.

Everything you need to be happy, healthy and at peace with your life can be found by living in the moment. It's only when we get stuck in the past or become fearful or anxious about the future that our happiness disappears.

Living in the moment is a great place to be and all it takes is to practice being mindful of your thoughts, feelings, and bodily sensations in the present moment. It has the power to give you space to gain new understandings and let go of those parts of you that cause suffering or struggle... and by the way grab this free guided meditation series to see how it works in practice.
www.MasterYourMindspace.com/meditationprogram

THE POWER OF CHOICE

Becoming the Inner Smile

You may have heard the old saying, "Laughter is the best medicine." Did you know that when you laugh deeply and fully, in those moments every cell of your body is filled with happiness and health, unlike those times when laughter is absent from your life.

When did your sense of humor begin to disappear? Was it around the same time that "serious" attitudes started to assert themselves?

One day a lady at one of my workshops confided, "I used to be miserable all the time because I took life so seriously. My health suffered, my relationships were in ruins, and I couldn't remember the last time I had a good laugh."

As I drove home that evening and pondered this comment, I was reminded that the absence of happiness and laughter does indeed have a far reaching impact. I could not recall how often in the past I had subjected myself to bouts of self pity brought on by some circumstance or other. I have since learned the value of a smile a day, both within and without.

It is not hard to fill your inner and outer world with pleasure. The reasoning is simple. If you can be taught to judge your life then you can also teach yourself to value it. The inner smile comes when you live fully with power and awareness.

Entraining your mind to value life means making happiness a choice. Just the same as you choose what you are going to eat or wear during the day, you can also make choices regarding joyful living.

This does not mean that you have to isolate and protect yourself from the world in order to be at peace. It means that you find a way to accept both your strengths and weaknesses with the same love and understanding.

Then there are no more enemies to conquer and you will always be victorious. Happiness and joy are an integral part of your existence and are always with you, regardless of how cleverly your mind may conceal this fact from you.

There are two types of happiness. One comes from the pleasurable experiences of life around you, the other comes from the experience of life lived in harmony within you. One is temporary and subject to change, the other is permanent and unshakable.

Happy To Be Here

Right now, in this moment you can choose to experience how it feels to be happy right here, right now for no reason at all.

Happiness is a way of life, not a destination

The fastest way to have more happiness is to connect with your body. It's quite a challenge for people who live in their head to really be happy because they are constantly analyzing and interpreting data, which leaves little space for peace and calmness.

HERE'S HOW TO SPEND THE NEXT 5 MINUTES

Start by closing your eyes and make sure that your body is comfortable. Now take several slow, deep breaths through your nose and down into your belly and then slowly and gently exhale out your mouth.

As you do this, focus on letting go of any tension in your body with each breath out. Imagine it being released from your body through your breath out. Continue to do this for five minutes, moving deeper and deeper into a relaxed state.

Then when you are ready open your eyes and see how you feel. What do you notice about your mind and body? If you allowed yourself to really relax, then your mind will quiet and your body will be energized.

This whole process takes just a few moments, yet the benefits are enormous. If you are truly relaxed your happiness will instantly appear as a warm, fuzzy feeling throughout your body. Then you are free to tap into this depthless well of joy whenever you choose.

Choose It - or Lose It

I know from years of experience that the power of choice shapes our future and determines who we are now and what we can have, and be, in the future.

Many times people say things like, "I would like to make more money", or "I'd like to get along better with my family", or "I'd like to do something really worthwhile with my life." These types of statements are not commitments to action. They are merely expressions of interest.

Being interested in changing your life and being committed to changing it are two entirely different matters. One is based on hope and is basically powerless to create change in your life, while the other supplies you with the power you need to launch into your next project.

Being committed to achieving the highest quality of life you can have is a lifelong endeavor of personal satisfaction. It does not have to be hard work. That too is a choice. The standards that you set for yourself when committing to anything you want to achieve must never falter, no matter what.

Even if you become despondent, you lose your job, or your family disowns you, the economy crashes, even if rain or fire, wind or earth wreaks havoc upon you, never lose sight of where you are going and who you want to be when you get there.

Joyful Living

I have found that the most valuable things in life come quietly and simply.

Simplicity is the master key to joyful living.

Until you understand and appreciate that you will continue to struggle through life, attempting to prove to yourself and the universe that you are only worthy of happiness when you have climbed the next imaginary mountain.

After all, do you remember as a child hearing statements like, "Things have been so good lately I wonder when something bad is going to happen?", or "You must work long and hard to get what you want."

These are only two examples of a multitude of beliefs that need to be replaced with constructive and empowering thought patterns that will prove to you that joyful living is your birthright.

I will define joy as the following sensations:

- Happiness
- Pleasure
- Peace
- Relaxation
- Abundance

- Harmony
- Positive Emotions
- Balance
- Well Being
- Passion

Joy allows your mind, body, and spirits to be uplifted, while misery and stressful living brings heaviness and hardship. No one in their right mind would consciously choose misery, yet the fact remains that it is a huge part of many people's lives.

This is why it is so important to make happiness a choice. Choose to resolve problems instead of whining about them. Change your attitude towards negative experiences, and embrace all your emotions equally. You will soon develop powerful new belief systems that will cause your self-esteem to come alive and joyful living to become a way of life.

Misery or unhappiness consists of experiences like:

- Fear
- Anger
- Blame
- Pain
- Failure
- Suffering
- Confusion
- Disharmony
- Negativity
- Neurosis

Keep these things in mind and understand that the quality of your life and the amount of happiness you can experience at any given moment is directly related to whether you are focusing on misery or joy.

Remember also that happiness or misery can never happen in the future - they always happen NOW.

Lightening the Load

Connecting with your authentic self is vital to understanding the relationship between what you have and what you want. There are no secrets or mysteries to life, only knowledge. The more knowledge you have about yourself, the less inclined you will be to judge, criticize or blame anything outside of you for your misfortunes.

Moving forward with confidence, courage, and trust are important elements in embracing self discovery. One of the things that limits this discovery is carrying around excess baggage from the past. Most of the time, this baggage doesn't even belong to you, yet it persists in coming along for the ride anyway.

This baggage comes in many forms. Sometimes, it is carried as beliefs you have borrowed from the family, friends, or society that helped condition your mind from birth. Other times it is deeply buried emotional experiences that created a wound that has never properly healed.

Some of the belief systems that you carry around with you as excess baggage may look like:

- Money buys happiness

- It is selfish to consider yourself before others

- If you're not nice to others you won't be liked

- If you don't do as you're told you will be punished

- Relationships are painful

- Emotions are never to be displayed in public

- You are responsible for the feelings of others

- Life is not meant to be easy

- Men/women can't be trusted

- Children should be seen and not heard

- What you have to say is not important

Regardless of where your baggage comes from, it can be released. By identifying the thought patterns that you give power to in your life, you can begin the process of changing them.

HERE'S HOW TO SPEND THE NEXT 5 MINUTES

Take a moment now to write down some of the obvious beliefs that you are carrying around as excess baggage. Take your time and be aware of any feelings that come up for you. Do nothing but watch any thoughts or feelings you are experiencing and continue with your list.

When you have finished the list fold it neatly a few times, write your name on the back of it, and then burn it. Fire symbolizes cleansing. This demonstrates to your subconscious mind that you are cleansing it of past limitations and starting your life from this moment on with a clean slate.

Do this technique as often as you like. Remember, though, that you must still take the actions that reinforce how you want your life to be to feel the full benefits.

Mass Hysteria

Look around you in the world and notice the limiting perceptions of life that are being reinforced every day by people, the media, advertising, business, and society in general. How many of these perceptions contain negativity or are based on fear, misery, violence, paranoia, chaos, or destruction?

You are constantly absorbing this information deep within your mind and body, and this accumulates as part of your excess baggage.

What beliefs do you have that you can say belong wholly to you, or are you just mimicking the borrowed beliefs of the world around you? Knowing *your* truth is a vital part of discovering who you are and what you want out of life.

Living your life through, or for others, is easy to do but rarely leads to fulfillment. Rather, it fosters an attitude of sacrifice and denial that inevitably leads to resentment and unhappiness.

To know what your truth is with regard to any person, place, or circumstance, you must first weed out what does not belong to you. A good example of this happened for me as I was about to finish high school.

My father wanted me to be a pilot in the Air Force. I, on the other hand, had no idea what I wanted to do. In order to play the game, I went along to a career guidance day and after spending the entire day looking at various career paths, I left feeling more confused than ever.

Deep in my heart I knew that I did not really want to think about a fulltime career yet, but I did not have the courage to express this. As the years went by I wandered from one meaningless job to the next. It took twelve years of frustration and disillusion before I finally gave myself permission to live my dreams.

There's no point blaming your parents, society, or education for the way your life may be right now. Instead, turn your gaze inward and take the time to get to know who you are, what you really want, and how you can go about attaining it.

Flexibility Brings Sensibility

Whatever is true for you in one moment must be open to negotiation in the next otherwise you will never find consistent happiness.

Truth can be expressed as:

- Your opinion

- The opinions of others

- Your feelings

- The feelings of others

- The facts according to you

- The facts according to others

- Reality (what *is* happening)

Even if other people remain steadfast in their opinions, as long as you allow yourself to remain open and available to change, you will become a greater person.

Having inflexible beliefs or attitudes is like trying to use a steel cable to tie up your shoelaces. Imagine if a devout Christian and an atheist were locked in a room for several hours together to talk about their beliefs. What do you think would happen?

What if everyone went around saying, "I am right and you are wrong," to everyone else they came across.

What hope would there be for peace, joy, and harmony then? By allowing others their truth and at the same time not compromising your own integrity, you take a major step up in empowered living.

Let me ask you this question. How did you feel the last time someone rejected, judged or invalidated your point of view on something?

There are numerous situations in your day to day lives and your interactions with people where you will find this happening. One of the most obvious places is with those closest to you such as your loved ones or workmates.

These relationships are your greatest opportunity for growth because they show you things about yourself that you would rather the world didn't know. It is this exposure that can become your greatest testament to personal development. If you learn to love the parts of you that you avoid the most your self-esteem will skyrocket.

Not many people acknowledge their partners for being a brilliant teacher to them. However, as you develop an attitude of gratitude towards all that life brings you, not only will your self-esteem increase, so too will your appreciation for those that you attract into your life.

Just Is

Consider our legal system. It is based upon the perceptions of right and wrong. If there were no 'right' how could there be any 'wrong'? Therefore, perception in this instance is based upon comparison, which in turn creates judgment. The legal system is designed as a way to ensure justice through judgment of thoughts (intention) or behaviors.

In a metaphysical understanding, judgment of self and others is what prevents you from going beyond your ego limitations. Judgment is an acquired behavior.

If you've ever had a child you'll know that a baby does not come into the world judging life. A baby plays, laughs when it's happy, cries when it's sad, and lets you know the moment something is wrong. These are the things that you and I would be better off remembering instead of being critical of ourselves or others.

A baby does not know fear, yet it is in touch with its feelings. Such is the simplicity of an uncluttered mind. Eventually, the baby will be judged and in turn will learn to judge, but until that happens it is free to enjoy this gigantic playground it has been born into.

Here's a challenge for you.

Over the next 24 hours try not to say or do anything that is judgmental towards others.

This does not mean that you can't set boundaries and remind others when they have crossed the line. You must do this to stay emotional healthy and feel safe and secure within yourself.

Instead, if you find yourself having judgmental thoughts about someone, either walk away until you can talk with them calmly or say nothing at all.

No Blame, No Shame, No Pain!

You could, and many people often do, spend a lifetime blaming others for past experiences, or present circumstances. Blame is a game of passing the buck.

It means that you are not willing to take responsibility for what is happening within your mental, physical, or emotional world. As soon as you decide that "the buck stops here", you can count on becoming free from guilt, regret, judgment, and pain.

It is amazing how quickly issues resolve themselves when you put this wisdom into practice. Blame is like a disease that eats away inside you if you let it. Blame ultimately affects the quality of your life and those around you.

It is a childish game that serves no purpose other than to let life know that having a temper tantrum is far more important to you than creating peace and happiness.

You may have spent time at seminars, counseling, or other therapies but what does it really take to allow you the peace of mind to get on with your life in joy? You could do it right now if you wanted to.

In the spectacular Walt Disney movie, "The Lion King", young Simba finds himself being smacked on the head with a bamboo cane by a somewhat eccentric, yet wise old monkey. When Simba asks, "What did you do that for?" The wise monkey replies, "What does it matter, it's already in the past."

When you are ready, willing and able to let go of the past, the present will be there to greet you like the sun rising up over the horizon, bringing with it the promise of new life and adventure.

My motto is to forgive and forget. It is not hard to do when you want to create the best life possible for yourself, and those you love. While you are stuck in the past, you are not free to explore the grandeur of where you are now.

I have counseled enough people to know that forgiving and forgetting is the last thing that some people are interested in. No matter what your life has been like up until now, unless you can find a way to get over past issues, then difficulties will plague your path.

The simplest and most effective way to "bury your dead" and enjoy a peaceful life, is to focus your mind, body, and emotions in the present moment.

Whether you are shopping, eating, cleaning, working, meditating, or driving a car, allow yourself to become fully alive to the sensations that are happening within and around you - all it takes is awareness. This will bring your attention powerfully into the present moment and then you will be filled with an abundance of life now.

Approval Rating

How often do you notice that you are either seeking approval from others, or they are seeking it from you?

Approving of yourself means that whatever you want to do is good enough for you, even if others do not agree. Approving of others means that whatever they want to do is good enough for them, even if you don't like it.

During my teen years I developed a mammoth-sized crush on a girl called Susan, at my school. We shared only one class together and naturally that was my favorite. From the moment I saw Susan, I was a mess.

My days revolved around seeing Susan from a distance, any chance I got. I would walk past her house after school, just on the off chance that I would get a glimpse of her.

Unfortunately, Susan never even knew that I existed. I was unable to muster up the courage to approach her, except in my mind. Every time I got near Susan, I became a quivering mass of jelly, my mind turned to mush and suddenly my legs wouldn't move. The girl of my dreams went from one boy to the next and all I could do was watch.

Looking back on this teen drama, I can see where non-approval of myself lumbered me with self-judgment and fear of rejection. I was so paralyzed by these things that there never was any chance of us getting together, even if Susan had been interested.

Approving of your self is a big deal. Without self-approval you are at the mercy of those that either will, or won't, give it to you. Your choices become limited, your self-worth becomes questionable, your fears become larger, and your world becomes smaller. All of these things and many more are a part of the burden that comes with seeking approval from the outside.

When you love and approve of yourself you no longer need validation from the world around you – then you will know a tremendous peace inside you.

For now, focus on approving of yourself first and foremost before you go out of your way to be a hero to others.

Let your wants, needs and desires be important enough to have priority in your life. When you have given goodness to yourself, then let it flow freely from you. You will be amazed at the difference in the quality of your life.

HERE'S HOW TO SPEND THE NEXT 5 MINUTES

Close your eyes and repeat this statement to yourself, "I love and approve of myself and I feel...........". The words that follow "I feel" is whatever comes into your mind at the time. Do this for five minutes and let whatever is true for you be okay.

For example, I might start off with, "I love and approve of myself, and I feel hungry". Then the next statement might be, "I love and approve of myself, and I feel distracted". And so you go on, not limiting how you feel or what's going on for you. This is a very powerful exercise because you are sending a powerful message to yourself that everything about you is okay. This is the way to drop judgment from your mind and live a live a life of love and acceptance.

The Key to Self Approval

When you truly love and approve of yourself then your life will rapidly heal from the inside-out. Any stress, worries, or anxieties you may have had will melt away and in their place you'll find a deeper calmness and contentment than ever before. Choose one of the statements below or make up your own and repeat it over and over again in your head for at least five minutes a day until it becomes true for you.

- I AM OKAY - no matter what.

- I love and approve of myself - all the time.

- Within me is a powerhouse of love to share.

- I forgive myself for holding on to past pains.

- I am worthy of living in JOY.

- I understand that my past has given me the strength I needed to become who I am now.

- I release the past and live fully NOW.

RELEASING SELF SABOTAGE

A Heart Act to Follow

What is self-sabotage? Self-sabotage is literally a cry for help. It happens when you least expect it and influences your conscious and subconscious mind.

Self-sabotage can look like:

- Resistance to change

- An accident

- Illness

- Poverty

- Guilt

- Excuses

- Pain

Self-sabotage literally means cutting off your nose to spite your face. No rational or sane person would do such a thing, yet no one said our unconscious mind was either of those things.

Many things happen to us as we go through life. Most of the trauma and pain we suppress is stored in our subconscious mind and energetically in our body as repressed emotions.

When an outer experience triggers emotional reactions within us, quite often this opens the floodgates to our past. Then the energy of those experiences is released into our physical world and that's when you can expect the unexpected.

There are countless times each day that you are sabotaging your happiness and joy. Even a thought like, "Gosh, things have been going so well lately, I wonder when something bad is going to happen?" can be a trigger that calls forth an illness, accident, or unexpected disaster into your life.

Paul, a good friend of mine, came with me one Sunday afternoon to a local swap meet. Soon after arriving, he came upon an electric guitar that he liked. The price was a bargain; it was in magnificent condition and he immediately fell in love with it. However, I watched as he put the guitar down and said to the seller, "I will think about it for a moment".

About five minutes later, as we were standing in front of another stall, my friend turned to me and asked, "Do you think I should buy the guitar?"

"What is in your heart?" I asked.

A childlike grin appeared on his face and he hurried off to purchase his prize. Within a few moments my friend returned, looking glum and disappointed. He told me that the guitar had just been sold and he was upset with himself for procrastinating over it.

This bugged my friend for over two weeks. I can't remember how many times I heard Paul call himself an idiot because he didn't buy the guitar on the spot.

This is a great lesson in self-sabotage. If you are carrying around beliefs that you are not worthy to have what you desire, or you allow your mind to argue with your heart, then self-inflicted suffering will come your way.

Most of our inner conflicts come from lack of self-worth and our self-sabotaging beliefs are the power behind the lack.

My friend had not been expecting to find anything that he wanted, so he had been thrown off balance. He had allowed himself to become confused and indecisive. His indecision cost him his heart's desire.

Even indecision or uncertainty can be a self-sabotaging tendency that keeps you stuck in your head, and closed to your heart. Then, like a child whose favorite toy was taken away from it, you will grieve over your loss.

All limiting belief systems come from the past. The key is to recognize how they serve you (what you get out of them) in your daily life. Are they allowing joy and balance, or are they creating fear and misery?

The first step in the process of releasing self-sabotage is to recognize when it is happening.

Recognizing Self Sabotage

The normal state of balance for a person is a peaceful mind, healthy body, and relaxed emotions. A self-sabotaging belief system is identified by becoming aware of any mental, physical, or emotional imbalances you may be experiencing.

At any time that you feel confused, frightened, angry, nervous or uncertain, you can be assured that you are at the edge of a limiting belief system. This is what causes discomfort in your life.

By recognizing the boundaries of your beliefs you can choose to expand beyond them by not reacting to them and thereby taking away their power to sabotage your happiness and joy. Most importantly, peace of mind will guide you safely through any turbulence of the past.

As soon as you recognize a self-sabotaging belief system, you can take whatever action is necessary to turn it into a "self-supporting" belief.

The great news is that this can be done quite easily and simply. You have already been given plenty of tools to assist you in this and there are plenty more to come.

Imagination - A Place of Becoming

Our imagination is one of the most powerful tools we have to enable us to explore broader horizons in our lives. We can use our imagination either constructively, to benefit us, or destructively, to limit us. For example, optimists use their imagination constructively, while pessimists explore the hardship of living.

If you can focus on solutions rather than problems you will reap the benefits of using your imagination to create a better life for yourself.

At one of my seminars, a young businessman approached me during a break and said, "I don't seem to have enough hours in the day to get all the things done that I want to do, and it's frustrating me to the point where I'm not sleeping properly at night. Can you suggest anything I might be able to do to change this pattern?"

I thought about his question for a moment and then replied, "You are focusing on the problem and not the solution."

A frown appeared on his forehead and after a moment he replied, "What do you mean?"

I said, "You are looking at what you don't have, which becomes a problem, rather than what you can do about it, which becomes a challenge."

A short time later I received a letter of appreciation from him, telling me that he had just completed a time management course.

As a result of doing the course he was now more productive than ever, slept peacefully at night and had more than enough time to do everything he wanted to do.

You can also use your imagination to resolve past conflicts. Nothing more is required than a little time and a quiet place to reflect.

Unresolved issues always have emotional energy attached to them. This is what causes them to stay unresolved. If you can change the emotional charge you have towards the issue, then you will be able to forgive and forget, and get on with your life in peace.

HERE'S HOW TO SPEND THE NEXT 5 MINUTES

To begin the process of releasing the emotional charge, just use your imagination to re-create the scenario in your mind and then change the parts you didn't enjoy, to ones that you do. Imagine a scenario that has an ending that you would like to see happen, even if the real ending was disastrous.

This technique allows you to use your mind to begin to think of different ways to handle situations that you are not used to. Eventually, you will handle similar situations in the future in the way you are rehearsing in your mind. Then your conflicts will be resolved before they happen.

Agreeing - The Power to Win

When you find yourself involved in an unpleasant situation with another person, here is a simple technique that you can use - agree with them.

If someone thinks that Bugs Bunny should be made President of the United States, then what does it matter if you think it's a stupid idea or not? It costs nothing to say to them, "Sure, why not!" instead of trying to belittle them, or prove that you are right and they are wrong.

You can be much more effective in resolving conflict before it begins if you listen and communicate with people, rather than preach at them. By agreeing with their point of view, you validate them, and when that happens you both win. When you invalidate another person that is when the sparks fly.

Try telling a baby that it can't have its rattle back and watch what happens. No human being likes to be told "no", yet when you disagree with someone, that is what you are saying.

By saying "yes", you become a giver of life. People will respond to you with more respect and appreciation, as well as themselves feeling respected and supported. Relationships will blossom, self-worth skyrockets, and there is a whole new glow about you that will leave others bewildered and pleasantly surprised.

Agreeing with others does not mean becoming compliant or giving your power away to others to control you.

You can agree with someone while allowing yourself to be comforted by the truth that you know in your heart. As long as you are happy with what you know, that is all that really matters.

By validating someone else's point of view you are opening the door between you to make a connection based on acceptance, rather than judgment or criticism. This is the secret to having amazing relationships with everyone you meet or spend time with.

You can never force people to change their opinions or attitudes. The only time anyone will ever change is when they are ready. By being agreeable and letting others know that what they think and feel matters, you will matter to them.

HERE'S HOW TO SPEND THE NEXT 5 MINUTES

The next time someone says something to you that you would normally disagree with, instead see if you can find a way to express to them that they are right. Remember that whenever anyone says anything that from their point of view they are right, so it's really just a matter of looking at things from their point of view and letting them know that you get it. This will help everyone you communicate with to feel validated and accepted for who they are.

The Power of Words

Let us look at some of the words we constantly express to the world and what they create for us. Words can either add to the quality of your life, or detract from it. They have the power to bring great happiness and joy to your life and the lives of those around you, or be powerfully destructive.

There are also words that empower you, while others disempower you without you even knowing, just because of the hidden meaning they carry within them.

One of the fastest ways to have more control in your life and get what you want faster is to take charge of your words and the language you use.

The words you consistently use will ultimately shape the quality of your future.

Let's look at some examples of words that you can immediately change in your vocabulary to create a more confident and compelling future.

The first word is, can't (can-not). This word implies that you have no choice and that you are a victim. A more responsible word to use in its place is won't (will-not). Can't is a limitation. Won't is a choice.

The next word is, should. This word implies expectation of self or others. Expectation is not living in the present moment with awareness of what you desire in your heart. Whenever you find yourself using should, you are most likely coming from the point of view of obligation, rather than joy.

Should, often creates resentment, frustration, anger, and unhappiness. It creates limitation of what is possible for you to have, be and do and takes away your power to choose. Consider replacing *should* with *could*.

For example, 'I should wash the dishes, it's my turn' (obligation, expectation) and substitute; 'I could wash the dishes! This way you are choosing your destiny with power.

You will often hear people say to others, "You should do this," or, "You should do that". What nonsense! There is never anything that you should do, but there is a lot you could do if you chose to.

When someone tells you that you 'should' do something, then reframe it in your mind, or let them know that you 'could' do it if you wanted to.

This also applies to you. Don't put unreal expectations on others by telling them what they should do or how they should do it. Instead, help them to become more empowered by giving them a choice of what they could do, knowing that if they choose not to do anything, this is perfectly okay. It is their right to do so.

The word 'shouldn't' is a word that implies judgment of self or others. This word is fear based, carries a negative energy, and is not taking responsibility for what is happening, either within you or around you.

The best thing to do with this word is to make a choice as to whether you want to do something or not. This will give you a clear path to follow and give you back your power to be in control your life.

'Have to' is also another interesting phrase. This implies lack of choice and signifies issues of control, inflexibility, and expectations. Whenever you believe that you 'have to' do something or others have an expectation that you 'have to' do something, then substitute 'want to' in its place. 'Want to' allows choice and empowers your actions.

Another interesting word is 'try'. The meaning of this word implies success or failure is possible. It is non committal and non definitive. Consider replacing try with, I will. This carries a positive energy of choice that will enable you to take bigger steps towards your goals.

The next words are 'might' and 'maybe'. The energy of these words implies uncertainty, confusion, and avoidance. To affirm your willingness to participate in life with joy and certainty use the statement, "I choose".

Then there is 'but'. This word is often used as a negation in a sentence, or phrase, when you really mean 'no'. This word is also used as an excuse for not being honest about what you really want to do, or say. It limits your empowerment, and sends messages of lack of self-worth to the universe.

Replacing 'but' with 'and' will cause your energy to become more open, allowing, and creative. If you mean 'no', then say it. This was particularly gratifying for me to become aware of and it still keeps me amused as I watch others chasing their butts.

Take special notice of the words that you are using and constantly affirming to yourself, others, and the world.

Are they positive and reinforcing growth, harmony, joy, and life-giving tendencies? Or are they negative and reinforcing pain, misery, suffering, and life-destroying tendencies?

Here's a checklist of the words we just covered and what you can now replace them with to take more control of your emotions, actions and self confidence.

- Can't = Won't
- Should = Could

- Have to = Want to
- Try = I Will

- Shouldn't = I Choose
- Must = I Choose

- NO = NO
- YES = YES

- Might = I Choose
- Maybe = I Choose

HERE'S HOW TO SPEND THE NEXT 5 MINUTES

Choose one of the words from above that you are most keen to transform and then commit to using it consistently for the next seven days. Make a note in your journal describing what your experience was when you used the empowering word, instead of the old disempowering word.

This can include how you felt, what happened for the other person when you didn't give away your power or anything else you noticed

Express Delivery

Every word you express, the tone you use, the manner in which it is intended and the way it is received, carries energy to and from your body.

You are what you speak. If you speak, "I love my life!" then life agrees with you and sends you more to love. If you speak, "I hate my life!" then life also agrees with you and sends you more to hate – this is called the law of attraction.

On any given day, far too many words are spoken that have no real power or substance because there is little or no action taken to back them up. For example, if you make a commitment to do something and do not follow through, you are not honoring what you are saying.

When we become incongruent with what we say we want and the actions we take to achieve those goals, then we let ourselves down and end up becoming a quitter, rather than an achiever.

I recall when I was eighteen years old I dreamed and spoke of retiring at the age of thirty. It was when I turned thirty that I left my 9-5 job and started living my dreams. While I didn't retire from working, I did retire from doing work I hated and working for someone else and for me that is way better than retiring and waiting to die because you no longer feel needed or useful.

If you want to become greater than the sum of your past then before you speak or take action, stop for a moment and think about the consequences of what you do next. Make sure that what you put out is in alignment with your goals and values.

If you consistently speak words of kindness, and perform actions of compassion, then you will rarely experience anything other than absolute joy in your life.

Follow Your Heart

You are the only person who can change your life. No one else can do it for you, although there are some people who would like to believe they know what is best for you.

Whenever someone is attempting to convert you to their way of thinking, do your best to love them for whom they are, rather than judge what they do.

Listen attentively, for their opinion may be the same as yours. But if it's not, then be courageous enough to thank them for their opinion and follow your own heart's desire. Go with your own natural instinct, no matter how much opposition comes your way from so called do-gooders.

Act on the impulses or creative urges that inspire and excite you. Allow your choices to be swayed by happiness, rather than guilt or fear. When considering action, if your gut feeling says 'yes', then go with it. If it is 'no' then decline!

If you can do this at least once a day, you will be amazed at how uplifted you feel, how much energy you gain and how rapidly your life transforms for the better.

HERE'S HOW TO SPEND THE NEXT 5 MINUTES

Think about something that you have been putting off doing because you weren't sure of what you wanted to do. Now put your hands over your heart and with your eyes closed ask your heart what it wants. Then sit silently for a few minutes and just be aware of any thoughts, images, or feelings that may arise.

This is a very powerful exercise to do to begin re-connecting with your heart's desires and over time as you learn how it talks to you it will have a profound impact on the decisions you make and the quality of life you live.

BELIEF IT OR NOT

I'll See It, When I Believe It!

Imagine for a moment that you are standing on top of the highest mountain in the world. It is a clear sunny day and a brilliant blue sky stretches out before you like an endless ocean of water.

Now visualize that you are inside a small dark room. This room is not much bigger than your body. Even with your eyes open you are unable to penetrate the inky blackness that seems to permeate within and around you.

Which scenario best describes the quality of your life right now? Are you happy with your view of life or is there room for improvement?

Self improvement begins with opening the cupboard door and poking your head out. Who knows what you might find if you take a chance and explore beyond the world you already know.

When I first started taking risks to explore new areas of my life it was both frightening and exciting at the same time. I was never one to take small steps. For me it was more like gigantic leaps of faith. Sometimes I would land safely on my feet and other times I would be tossed around like salad in a bowl.

I am pleased to say that I survived all my adventures and misadventures and have absolutely no regrets about my past. The point is that you can sit back and watch life pass you by or you can take responsibility for generating a powerful future of happiness filled with everything you desire.

HERE'S HOW TO SPEND THE NEXT 5 MINUTES

You can start right now by buying a journal, or starting up a goals page and writing down a list of goals that you would like to attain over the next three months and twelve months. If you are married, have a family, or share your life with someone, then it might be fun to do this exercise together.

Write down some goals that are going to be easy to attain. Then throw all caution to the wind and let your imagination go. You may be amazed at the results.

Committing your goals to paper is a powerful step forward in creating them. The next step is to take action towards achieving those goals that require the least amount of time or effort.

By taking steps, even small ones, towards attaining your goals, you are declaring to your subconscious mind that you are a force to be reckoned with. The only time you won't get what you want is when you give up. Giving up is easy to do because it requires no effort. This is why so many people allow their dreams to fade away.

Once you prove to yourself that you deserve to have what you want, then you will be given all the energy you need to make it happen.

Sometimes a plan of action is a handy tool to use to map out exactly how you are going to complete your goal, especially at those times when you feel stuck. Then you can instantly refer to the plan and get back on track again.

You won't always need a plan. Often, things will happen as a series of apparent coincidences. When this happens, be assured that you are definitely on the right track and life is flowing in harmony with your desires. Be thankful for these times and acknowledge that you created this experience even if you have no idea how.

A Pleasant Surprise

Incredible things can and do happen all the time. If they are not happening in your life, then from this moment on, allow yourself to have at least one pleasant surprise a day. They are happening all the time. It's just that we don't always acknowledge them because we are too busy, too tired, too bored, or any number of other reasons.

As soon as you wake up each morning start the day by anticipating the arrival of your pleasant surprise. Then, let it go and remember to be prepared to acknowledge and appreciate it when it appears.

Mass Hysteria

Belief systems are not limited to your own personality. They can also belong to groups, cultures and the entire planet. An American friend of mine grew up believing that the Russians and communism were out to destroy world peace and democracy. One day he decided to visit Russia with a group of people and confront the enemy for himself.

His experience with Russian people reveaIed to him that they were just like you and me. They, too, wanted a peaceful life, to feed their children and also feared a nuclear holocaust.

My friend and his party were treated like honored guests. They were invited into homes for meals, taken on breathtaking tours of the countryside and shown that these people had the same hopes, fears, and emotions that we all share.

A few years later, the Russian government fell, the Berlin wall came down, and a new era dawned on world peace. There never was any threat to America or its people. The propaganda mechanism of militant minds needed to justify trillions of dollars spent annually on the arms race. What better way to ensure funding than through fear?

It never ceases to amaze me how much power the media has to generate mass beliefs. A carefully planned story can influence the minds and beliefs of an entire country in a single blow.

An example of a mass generated belief can be easily seen in how the media and tabloids portray the images of the ideal man and woman. These images reach deep into our subconscious mind and influence the way we think about ourselves and others.

While this is good business for the glamour magazines, weight loss centers, hairdressers, dentists, plastic surgeons and gymnasiums, it does little to change the subconscious beliefs that cause so many people to feel ugly and unimportant on the inside.

Self criticism is a disease that eats away your self-esteem from within. It literally consumes your power to be happy and leaves pain and misery in its wake.

Deep within you there is a place that is judgment free. Until you know that place from your own experience, self-judgment will continue to motivate you to chase illusions. One of these illusions is that you are not already perfect.

Who you are on the inside has, and always will be, absolutely perfect. The only imperfection belongs to what you think. You cannot think your way into perfection, but you can think your way out of it.

There is nothing wrong with changing your image on the outside. It can bring renewed confidence, power, and happiness. However, the most powerful changes happen when you work on both the inner and the outer. Then your transformation is more than just cosmetics - it is permanent.

A Mask a Day

In the same way that a police-officer puts on a uniform to create an image of authority, your life is filled with images that are created through the many masks of your personality.

In the outrageous film, "The Mask," Jim Carey discovers an ancient mystic mask that when worn, has the power to bring alive his inner fantasies and uninhibited personality. His normal timid temperament gives way to a deluge of devilish behavior, super-cool personality, and unbending flamboyance.

Although this portrayal takes us on a journey of extreme behavior, the symbology is quite accurate. Each day, you present many masks (identities) to the world that create an intricate dance between your ego personalities and the people and circumstances you interact with.

Are you the same person when you are with your mother, husband, children, boss, friends, or relatives? Or do you habitually alter your behavior depending on who you are with? What do you suppose causes these changes?

It is the relentless need for approval. As a child we learn to behave in certain ways in order to be accepted for who we are. It may not necessarily be a truthful representation of what we are feeling, thinking, or wanting to say and do, yet in order to fit in with the expectations of others we generally modify our behavior to be accepted.

This alone tells us that what we really fear is being powerful and authentic. Because we have never truly been accepted for who we are, this keeps our superficial personalities firmly wedged in place.

It is far more painful to keep avoiding yourself, than it is to relax and allow your authentic self to shine its brilliant light into the world. This part of you is abundantly filled with everything you need to enjoy a strong, healthy, peaceful, enjoyable, and fulfilling life.

On the other hand, your ego masks are masters of disguise, fear, and limitation. Which one would you choose to live if common sense prevailed?

These masks are not real. They belong to the world, not to you. If you can allow yourself to let your doubts and fears come and go without the need to change or avoid them, then you will experience the unlimited love of who you really are.

Underneath all your pains and fears exists a river of love that flows deep and strong within your heart. It is always there and once felt, can always be called upon, even in the darkest of moments.

Your mind is for the most part a creature of habit. It loves to focus on what is safe, comfortable, and known. This requires little effort because it is easy and doesn't require you to stretch beyond where you are.

Expanding your Mind Power will require a little stretching at first. Soon flexibility becomes a way of life and then your mind becomes a phenomenal tool for rapid and astounding growth.

I have counseled many men whose lives have been devastated by a breakdown in their marriage. Marriage is an identity. It creates the illusion of security, commitment, and love. When that identity changes then the illusion breaks down and your world is suddenly in chaos.

These things are always there, only now the mask is gone, as is the security blanket that it created. If you can stay with your fears, look them in the eye, and let them pass by without reacting to them, then the gaps that are created when an ego mask is released will be filled with love from the inside, where you exist in perfect harmony and joy.

When a person who smokes feels nervous, the tendency will be to light up a cigarette to calm their frazzled nerves. Instead, to overcome the mask of a smoker, you could stay aware of the feelings you are having and take your power back from the cigarettes by breathing slowly and deeply until your body and mind has relaxed.

Whenever you overcome a limiting habit in a supportive and empowering way, always remember to immediately reward yourself by doing something that brings you joy. This helps you to establish positive pathways of growth within your mind, body, and emotions.

What Makes Your Heart Sing

Your happiness and misery are directly connected to how much attention you give to an identity and whether you allow it to be a positive or negative experience.

The world is made up of millions of moving parts, and each part is important to the whole, no matter how trivial it may seem. There are people who sit in factories all day, repair automobiles, stamp packages, take money at toll booths, clean bathrooms, bury the dead, or even prostitute themselves to make a living.

These are just some of the things that my heart would not find joy in. They have no place in my life except that I am aware they exist and I honor whatever choices other people make to live in the world. In the past, I believed that I had to do things that I didn't like simply because my fears were stronger than my confidence.

Now, everything I do flows from my heart and inner bliss. Whenever I follow my joy, my heart sings with happiness. Best of all I no longer work for a living, I live what I love and it works for me!

Thy Will Be Done

During one of my eight-week workshops Elizabeth kept complaining about her husband's shortcomings. It was not that he was a bad person in any way. The main problem seemed to be that Elizabeth felt used and neglected.

After a while, I realized that Elizabeth was not interested in taking responsibility for her feelings, so I asked her what she was willing to do to allow her relationship to be more enjoyable.

Elizabeth was unable to come up with an answer. I suggested many possibilities to her, but I could see that her mind was not going to let this transformation be easy. Eventually, Elizabeth and her husband separated. That day, she came to see me. This time she was devastated and uncontrollably hysterical.

Several hours of intense emotional turmoil followed. Finally, through mental and emotional exhaustion, Elizabeth gave up the struggle, allowing her true feelings to be felt without blame. Afterwards, a deep calmness and quiet came over Elizabeth. Her face and body relaxed and she looked more peaceful and contented than I had seen her in quite some time.

From this place of peace and clarity, Elizabeth realized that her resentment and anger towards her husband stemmed from her low self-esteem that told her she was not worthy to be in a happy, fulfilled relationship. Her greatest fear was that her husband would leave her for another woman. Now this circumstance had eventuated, and the fear had to be faced.

Relief flooded through Elizabeth as she forgave herself for allowing her fears to control her life. Within a few months, Elizabeth had moved into her own place, started up her own home-based business and for the first time ever, was living by herself and enjoying her new found freedom, strength, and independence.

The greatest source of power in your life comes from the ability to be flexible enough to change your attitude towards your problems. Sometimes, we get so caught up in our ego masks, that every thought, emotion, and action is affected by them.

At these times you must do whatever it takes to free yourself from the chains of misery that you have wrapped around you.

If drastic action is required, then take it. If you are strong enough to change your attitude, then do it. If you have no strength at all, then find help. Most of all - *do something.* When the day finally comes that you are in harmony with all of your masks, chances are that you will no longer need them.

By recognizing the areas in your life that you are not enjoying, you can choose to do something about them, or choose not to do something about them. Either way, you win.

Anytime you choose the way your reality looks, you are being responsible. Then you are one step closer to knowing the truth of your inner self.

If you wish to stay miserable then have the courage to say, "I choose misery!" By doing this you are taking control of your life through making it a choice rather than being a victim of circumstance. Then, anytime you want, you can make a different choice to experience a different result.

There's No Paradise in Sacrifice

One day I awoke to the sound of my parents arguing. I was ten years old at the time and did not yet understand why parents acted the way they did. I had heard my parents arguing before, but never for so long, or so loud.

The air was filled with tension and as much as I tried to block out the noise by covering my ears with a pillow, it didn't help. When the arguing was over and the competitors had retired to their appropriate corners, my mother surprised me by coming into my room to talk to me.

My mother gingerly sat down on the edge of the bed, buried her head in her hands, and sobbed deeply for awhile. When she finally looked up at me and spoke she said, "I am going to leave your father"

I looked at her through the eyes of a ten-year-old child and said, "No you won't, mum."

"What do you mean?" my mother enquired.

"You have said that many times before and yet you are still here," I replied. My mother looked at me with genuine surprise before saying, "The only reason I stay here is for you children."

Many years later my mother confided to me that in my simplistic way I had seen right through her excuses. She realized that most of her life had been based on a lack of self worth to have, do, and be what she truly desired.

Sacrifice is the victim's way of justifying being miserable. When you lack self-esteem, the freedom to make choices is limited. You become bound by your inner critic who tells you what is right and what is wrong, regardless of what you really want.

There is never a good enough reason to put up with anything you don't enjoy. If you are 'putting up' with something in your life right now and you are justifying it out of a sense of obligation, guilt, fear, complacency, money, or any number of reasons, then you are just making excuses.

There is no excuse for unhappiness - only choice. When you make happiness a priority in your life then it's bound to happen.

Use every moment to focus on creating your dream life. Never lose sight of this vision, even if doubts appear. To give up your happiness for the sake of others is denying your right to live your life the way you want to.

The moment you are willing to accept nothing less than complete and absolute faith in yourself as a powerful being of love, then you can be all that you want to be, do all that you want to do, and have all that you want to have.

It is possible to be happy within the ego mask of sacrifice. The only time this happens is when you give unconditionally. That means you have no resentment towards what, when, how, why, or to whom you are giving. This is a pretty tall order for most people because resentment and blame work hand in hand with sacrifice.

When you no longer blame others for your own shortcomings then there is no need for resentment. And once you have let go of resentment in your life, then you are free from toxic relationships and causing yourself emotional distress that was doing more harm to you than good.

HERE'S HOW TO SPEND THE NEXT 5 MINUTES

Write down an area of your life that you still carry around resentment. As you write it down, let your emotions pour into the words you are writing. Do this for at least five minutes. This will help you to release it into the words you are writing. Then take that piece of paper and burn it. As you watch it burning, say out loud, *"I am so happy to be letting go of a part of me I no longer need."*

No More Limits

There are no limits to the amount of joy you can have in your life, except for the self-imposed ones. As much as we might like to think that others are responsible for what we do or don't have, the truth is that there is never a moment that goes by that we are not sealing our own fate.

Kathy came to see me regarding being tired, irritable and unhappy all the time. Kathy was fed up with being unwell and wanted some insight into what was causing her life to be so miserable. I asked Kathy to tell me when she was most unhappy during the day.

Kathy replied, "At work". I then asked her what sort of work she did and Kathy told me that she worked as a registered nurse.

"What do you enjoy the most about your work, Kathy?"

"Nothing, I hate it!" replied Kathy bitterly.

"What causes you to do something you hate?" I asked compassionately.

Kathy sighed and then with a forlorn look said, "It is the only way I know how to earn a living.

This was a big deal for Kathy. It took a lot of courage for her to look into the mirror of her life and go, "You know what? This doesn't work anymore. I want more out of my life than what I have now."

Kathy had been miserable at her job for years, but it wasn't until her physical body started letting her down that she finally recognized the need to do something about it. Now that Kathy was aware of what area needed changing in her life, she could do something about it.

Kathy's first choice was to leave her job. Almost miraculously her health improved overnight. As the days and weeks went by Kathy's fears of not being able to support herself proved to be unfounded.

Her happiness and laughter returned like a long lost friend and within one month Kathy was so inspired that she successfully started up her own home-based business.

Never underestimate the power that unhappiness has to influence the quality of your life. Always be prepared to look at yourself in the mirror and say, "Where can I allow more joy into my life now?"

Choosing Joy

Here's a really simple exercise to help you find more happiness and joy in your life:

HERE'S HOW TO SPEND THE NEXT 5 MINUTES

1. Identify where you are unhappy in your life.

2. Write down your answer (i.e. work, relationship, money, etc.)

3. Specify the cause of your unhappiness.

4.   Write down a plan of action (what you can do) to turn your unhappiness into joy. Be creative and seek advice if need be.

5.   Put your plan into action.

6.   If your plan is not working, change it.

7.   Do this every evening for seven days.

Bubble of Light

There comes a time when you start releasing unnecessary masks, effortlessly. These experiences are more energetic in nature than physical, yet their impact is enormous.

The closest analogy I can give you is the difference between a ripple in a pond and a tidal wave on the beach. A ripple gently reaches out over great distances, whereas a tidal wave releases all of its energy in one gigantic splash.

These times are heralded by sudden change that envelops you like an invisible bubble of light. Without warning you can be going about your daily life when suddenly, like a bolt of lightning out of the clear blue sky, your entire outlook on life shifts.

The first time this happened to me, I wandered around like a lost puppy for months. So sudden was the shift in my thoughts and feelings that it took quite some time to integrate what was happening to me.

My experience was pre-empted by a weekend "awakening" workshop. Afterwards, I recall sitting outside the main room, completely at a loss as to what to do next.

Instinctively I sought refuge with friends, family, and loved ones, yet all to no avail. I was stunned by the fact that no matter where I went or whom I was with, the emptiness and loneliness inside of me remained unchanged.

I felt completely isolated from the world by an invisible bubble that seemed to draw me deeper into a world that was new, yet in some way familiar.

Over the next few weeks and months, everything in my life radically changed without any apparent effort from me. It was like a part of me had been peeled away and the new me was yet to be realized.

Before I knew it I had a whole group of new friends, new interests, a business idea that I put into motion and even an entirely new way of connecting with people.

This is when I discovered that change is an ongoing part of personal growth. When you feel like the rug has been pulled out from under your feet, don't be too hasty to judge it. Instead, find the blessing that is being offered to you and enjoy whatever journey you are being guided to take.

These experiences only happen when some part of you is ready to receive them. For me, it was like being an infant once again. I had to learn a whole new way of being and in this there was great satisfaction.

When you give up struggling with your ego to cling to those parts of you that are no longer necessary, then life can expand within and around you with ease. All it takes to know when you have finished with something, be it a relationship, a job, a habit, or a way of life, is to trust your inner knowing and be aware of what your heart is telling you.

Change is the only constant in life. To resist it is to cause pain and to learn to flow with it brings peace and happiness.

WALKING YOUR TALK

Do what you say, say what you mean!

You learn more from the actions and behavior of those around you than you will ever learn from their words. If what you speak is to carry any meaning at all, it must be demonstrated by the actions you take.

Are you walking your talk? If not, you are giving mixed messages to those who share your life, especially your children. A child who grows up observing that what you say is not what you do learns that dishonesty is the best policy.

What did your parents' actions teach you about the meaning of love? Did you learn that love only works when people are happy, or did you learn that love can overcome all obstacles?

Children from broken homes learn that relationships don't last and love is painful. Why waste your breath telling a child that everything is okay, if your life is a mess?

Regardless of how well you might think that you are hiding your pain and frustration, a child instinctively knows when something is wrong. It is adults who have difficulty coping with truth, not children.

Children constantly bounce back from traumatic situations whereas adults often require years of therapy or medication. Children don't take life seriously until it is drummed into them that life is tough and people are not to be trusted.

For some of us, 'serious' attitudes happen the moment we get our first job. Then the reality of everyday living can be like an unexpected headache. For me, going to school was a breeze compared to the stress of entering the workforce.

Expectations run high, dreams come and go in the blink of an eye, and the search for fulfillment soon becomes forgotten as the need to survive takes over.

I certainly had my share of ups and downs in the workforce before experiencing the immense satisfaction of getting paid for what I love to do.

Never forget that everything you come across, be it a person, experience, or job you have, is an opportunity to have, be or do more with your life. There's no need to stay stuck in anything that you are not enjoying, especially those people or circumstances that you wish would go away. Typically, they are your grandest opportunity for growth.

You may not be able to see the light at the end of the tunnel from where you are standing but that doesn't mean it isn't there. As soon as you decide that you deserve to have a first class life, instead of a second-hand one, that's when the tide will start to turn in your favor.

Never underestimate your power to radically transform any part of your life instantly. All it takes is a decision to make a change and then follow through with that decision each and every day until it becomes a reality for you.

So many people tend to give up before they ever start to make a change because it can seem like an impossible task from where they are looking right now. Believe me, although it may seem to be easier to not take action, in the long run you will pay the ultimate price of letting yourself down.

That's why so many people turn to medication, gambling or addictive behavior. Their lives are so meaningless to them that they need to numb the pain by any means possible. This then harms the body or becomes a destructive force in their life, which results in more pain and suffering.

It takes courage to do what's right for you especially when you are not being supported by others. The great news is that for every step forward you make with courage, each step that follows gets easier and your courage gets stronger until eventually you become invincible in your resolves.

If that sounds good to you, then muster up whatever courage you need today to step toward the future you imagine for yourself and don't look back until you arrive. Yes, there will be obstacles but the way through them is to stay focused on your destination and that will keep you steady as you navigate whatever challenges pop up.

HERE'S HOW TO SPEND THE NEXT 5 MINUTES

Do something spontaneous and childlike for the next five minutes. Just imagine that you are an innocent child again and drop any ideas of being serious. Instead, let your inner child go free just for a few minutes and see what comes up. If you allow just five minutes a day to become playful and free-spirited, you may find yourself feeling younger and more alive again.

Accept Yourself

A friend of mine came to see me the other day, deeply disturbed by her emotional outburst during a class she was teaching.

"What is it about this incident that disturbs you?" I asked Vicki.

"I feel ashamed that I did not control my emotions and that I let my students see me that way," Vicki replied.

To many of us, it is not okay to express those parts of our lives that we do not understand. Angry outbursts often leave you feeling guilty for what you said or did, and then you feel bad about yourself.

There is nothing wrong with any feeling you have. There is also nothing wrong with expressing these feelings, if you do not judge them. It is the judgment of your behavior that causes the pain, not the actual experience. I have found that people often learn a great deal from a comment or two made in anger or frustration.

As soon as it's okay with you that you are angry, then it will be okay with others. Practice allowing yourself to express with feeling, and let go of the need to beat yourself up about it.

Valuable lessons can be learned even from those experiences that we judge the most. If you are unable to forgive or forget any aspect of your past, you might want to ask yourself, "Where am I stuck in pain and judgment?"

Consider the many different people who are a part of your life, from those you know intimately to those you hardly know at all. This includes people at your local bank, supermarket, neighbors, friends, relatives, and so this list goes on. How many of these people express themselves openly?

What is it that causes people to hold back expressing their truth? The answer is - fear. Fear of not being approved of, or accepted. The only person you ever need to be concerned about accepting you is you.

When you love and approve of yourself
regardless of the opinions of others,
then you are on the path to true freedom.

There is a simple and effective method of expressing yourself in a way that allows you to take full responsibility for your feelings and release the need for blame. This is to use statements like:

- "I am feeling (emotion) right now"
- "At this moment I feel (emotion)" or,
- "I feel (emotion)"

113

These statements allow you to retain your power by not projecting blame or justifying yourself. They are statements of fact. They keep your expressions empowered and truthful.

When someone says to you, "I feel confused" then there is no room for argument or debate. You are not being asked for an opinion, nor is one being given. It is a fact. Disagreements only eventuate when your need to be right, approved or accepted, is more important than honesty and responsibility.

While you were growing up, how many people taught you that the most important thing you can do is approve of yourself? And the reason this most likely didn't happen for you is because your role models never had that told or taught to them.

This means we grow up with a deeply buried belief that at some level we are not okay. Then this becomes a relentless driving force in our lives that leads us down paths constantly needing to be approved. The downside when we don't get this approval is that we either get resentful or feel like crap.

This is so easy to reverse if you are ready to let it go forever. All it takes is for you to constantly remind yourself that you are okay, no matter what.

For many years I used an affirmation where I constantly reinforced to myself that "I am okay, I am just feeling (something)", or "I am okay, I am just experiencing (whatever)." The important part was that I was retraining my mind to be okay no matter what I was thinking or feeling.

If this resonates with you, then by all means go ahead and use it yourself. It is very powerful and works like a dream but you must be consistent and repeat it all the time to yourself, especially when you are freaking out.

Some of the ways that we are not okay and try and put the blame for this onto others is when we make statements like:

- "You MAKE me so mad!"
- "What's WRONG with you?"
- "How could YOU do this to me?"

Can you see how these statements are focused on blame? By expressing yourself in this way you give away the power of your life to be forever manipulated by circumstances outside of you.

To overcome this self-sabotaging behavior just start expressing yourself with a more truthful awareness by using transformational vocabulary like, "I feel (emotion) when you...", and leave it at that. No justification for your behavior, no excuses for your actions and no projecting blame onto them for how you are feeling. In this scenario you end up the winner because you are taking responsibility for your experience.

The ABC of Stress Release

Your emotions cannot be told when they can and can't appear. They have an intrinsic life of their own that weaves its way into your daily life whether you like it or not. They often come when you least expect it and almost always when it is most inconvenient.

The key to moving through these turbulent times is to use simple and effective techniques to remind you to let go of any unpleasant feelings. The most effective tool that I have come across that allows instant results is your breath.

Take several slow, deep breaths, in through the nose and out through the mouth, the moment you become aware of any negativity within you. The word 'emotion' comes from the word 'emote' which means to 'move energy'. That's what your breath can and does do when it's allowed to do its job of clearing negative energy from your body.

To help with this process, ensure that you breathe all the way down into your lower belly area. Keep your spine as straight as possible, shoulders relaxed and your belly soft. When releasing your breath, let it out as slowly as possible.

If you do this technique correctly, you will find that by about the seventh or eighth breath you will be feeling calmer and your mind clearer.

By this stage your mind is clearer, your body is more relaxed and your capacity to handle any issues is greater – that is, if any issue still remains.

Here's what the ABC stands for in this technique.

- **A** = ACKNOWLEDGE - What you are feeling
- **B** = BREATHE - Slowly and deeply several times
- **C** = CHOOSE - Your behavior

This technique may sound simple and it is. Breathing is natural, convenient and, best of all, provides immediate relief.

This is a great key to pass on to others and you will be amazed at the feedback you get from those who choose to use it.

HERE'S HOW TO SPEND THE NEXT 5 MINUTES

Make sure you are seated comfortably in your chair, or you can stand if you like and then put your hands on your belly, close your eyes and breathe in slowly through your nose until you feel your breath connecting to your hands as your belly rises.

Then, slowly let your breath gently trickle out of your mouth until it has all been released. Then repeat this method several more times. The key here is to control your breathing in a slow and rhythmic way. Your hands stay on your belly the entire time so as to remind you of where your breath needs to go each time you breathe in.

Grab this free guided meditation series to see how it works in practice.

www.MasterYourMindspace.com/meditationprogram

Reflections of Nature

It is so easy to find beauty in nature. The magnificent colors, shapes, fragrances, sounds and images effortlessly fill our senses with joy and amazement. How easy it is to stare in awe at a giant redwood tree, or have your breath taken away by a dazzling sunset.

This beauty is apparently much more difficult to find in human beings. You would not think about taking a tree to court for falling on your car, but if another person dented it you might. If a massive earthquake destroyed your hometown and everyone in it, except for you, would it matter to the earthquake if you went insane with rage at it?

Does nature care if you spend years in therapy to overcome personal trauma? Not in the least. The earthquake did what it was meant to do and then vanished. Your traumas have nothing to do with the earthquake except that it provoked certain feelings within you.

The same applies to other people and experiences. The difficulty of forgetting about the actions of others comes from your ego's need to avoid taking responsibility for your feelings.

Remember, no one or no-thing can make you feel anything that you don't want to. You choose what feelings you have, even if they are in response to external triggers you always get to choose how you react to them. The choice may be unconscious, yet it still belongs to you. You also have one hundred percent control over how you choose to behave in response to your emotions.

There are many actors that have to do this each day. They arrive at their studio, or on location, change into their costumes and then slip into their appropriate character role. The greatest actors are those who can emotionalize the character they are portraying.

To do this they may need to get in touch with the same emotion inside of themselves, yet because they are not 'reacting' to an outside provocation they can turn their feelings off and on at will.

Your feelings belong to various ego identities that collectively make up your personality. It makes sense then that you should theoretically be able to call on any one feeling, or a variety of them, to come out and play any time you like. This tells us that emotions do not have to control us. Rather, that the opposite is true; we can take charge of them.

You will continue to be provoked into emotional upheaval by the world around you, until you decide that you only want to find the beauty in life, rather than the beast. When you no longer judge your feelings and you are at peace with even the most painful ones, then your life will reflect this beauty both on the inside and outside.

Normally emotions are triggered by other people or circumstances. Start to look at these people and circumstances as opportunities for growth. They can become your inspiration, rather than your enemy. If you pay attention to the messages they bring, you will discover where you are stuck in judgment.

The moment you relax and let go of the judgment through your breath, you will gradually become less reactive (unconscious) and more responsive (conscious) to the world around you. The benefits of this are enormous, the most profound being a life of peace and joy.

Within you there is a quiet respect for the power and beauty of nature, despite any tragedies that happen. Take this respect and apply it to human nature, no matter how much you are provoked. Find a way to see the beauty in all experiences and you will come to know your inner beauty.

If You Don't Mind, It Won't Matter

You have approximately fifty thousand thoughts per day, either consciously or subconsciously. Each of these thoughts has an energetic charge to it. Positive thoughts carry a positive charge and negative thoughts carry a negative charge. But until you obsess over, speak, or take action on any thought they have no real power.

Your life is shaped by your thoughts.
You become what you think about most
of the time. Think thoughts of peace
and happiness will follow.

Thoughts are like clouds in the sky. They will just float on by not disturbing you unless you get attached to them. Once this happens, then they can either turn into a raging storm, or cause you to laugh, dance, and sing.

Too much stress and anxiety in life can make it near on impossible for some to even imagine having a calm mind and relaxed body. That's when your head can feel like it's going to explode and your entire mind-body system goes into overload mode.

These are the times that it's even more critical to take time-out and slow down, even if just for a few minutes to de-stress and clear your head.

There can be no happiness or peace in your life if you don't learn how to quiet your mind.

A clear mind is the answer to a happier, healthier, and more enjoyable life.

HERE'S HOW TO SPEND THE NEXT 5 MINUTES

This is an exercise in clearing your mind. The first part is to focus your mind. To help with this make sure you are sitting comfortably. Then, put your left hand out in front of you and rest it palm upwards on something that supports it. This might be on your lap, or desk, or whatever is convenient.

Close your eyes and focus all your attention on the palm of your hand. You may be able to start to feel a warmth or tingling in the center of you palm as you do this. If any thoughts or feelings come along to distract you just remind yourself to come back to focusing on your palm.

Do this for five minutes and then sit quietly for a moment and just notice what is happening in

your mind and body. If you have managed to keep your focus on your palm your mind will now be clear and your body will be calm and relaxed.

UNCONDITIONAL LOVE

*The Key to Happy, Healthy, and Intimate
Relationships*

Love is one of the most overused and least understood words in any language. What you and I have been taught to believe is love has more to do with what we see, feel, and do, rather than a state of being. Being in love is intoxicating. It has no rhyme or reason to it and it transcends time and space.

Purity and innocence are the keys to unconditional love. You can find examples of this abundantly displayed in your pet dog. For example, have you noticed how enthusiastic and happy your dog is to see you each time you come home?

Does this resemble the treatment you give or get from other people? Yet we are supposed to be the intelligent creatures. What does this suggest to you about the relationship between love and intelligence?

If pets can live with such consistent joy and forgiveness, then surely it's possible for a human being to become exhilarated towards life again. Perhaps all that is really needed is to stop analyzing our lives and get on with enjoying them.

At another of my seminars an endearing man named John stood up and told us of how he had found love amidst pain.

"My wife has just left me, but I realized I left my wife a long time ago," John confessed.

"Looking back on the last few years," John continued, "I can see how I ignored my wife's needs and pretended that everything was okay between us. My life was about achievement and work. It never dawned on me that I was ignoring the most valuable part of my life until it was too late!"

John's voice was filled with emotion and the tears that welled in his eyes once might have embarrassed him, but now enabled him to see clearly.

The group was mesmerized by John. Everyone wanted to hear more.

"During the last few weeks I have had a lot of time to evaluate what I really want out of life. I realized that I had been putting self-importance before love. Now I have made a commitment to put love first - all the time, and practicing this vow has already changed my life." John's sincerity was touching everyone deeply.

"As for my relationship with my wife", John added, "I am not sure what the future holds but I know that whatever happens I am a new man and for that I feel immense gratitude."

The ability to see the road ahead is as easy as watching where you are going. If you wish to soar to new heights within yourself and with those you love, open your heart and remember to let love flow in and out whenever you can.

Slow and Steady Wins the Race

We live in an era of fast food, fast cars, fast relationships, and hectic lifestyles. Uncertainty and haste keep us running around in circles, never seeing the forest for the trees.

Is life passing by you so fast that you are forgetting to enjoy the journey? Don't wait for a 'wake-up' call to happen or a loved one to leave you before you slow down enough to appreciate what you already have.

If life is passing you by too fast then practice slowing down. For one hour, one day, one week or however long you can, consciously choose to slow down and enjoy the richness of the moment. Start by noticing what activities you are rushing to and from. When you become aware of haste then stop for a moment and have a few moments time-out.

If you still have a taste for haste, then allocate a special time each day to rush around. When we are aware of what we are doing and give ourselves permission for it to be okay then we are honoring our self as best we can.

Overcome the damaging impact of stress-related syndromes by slowing down and enjoying where you are. By making this a conscious decision you will win the race - even though there really is none. Slowing down doesn't mean becoming a blob. It means to walk slower, talk slower, listen more, eat slower, feel more, think less, and be in the world instead of dancing around it.

HERE'S HOW TO SPEND THE NEXT 5 MINUTES

Take time-out. Get up slowly from your chair and with awareness of each step you take, go outside and feel the warmth of the sun on your skin, the wind upon your face and skin, or simply go for a short stroll to give yourself space to connect with the outdoors and the movements and sensations that your body is experiencing.

It's great to take time-out on a regular basis, especially if you are stuck behind a desk all day. Ideally, you'd have a five minute break every hour and at the very least every 90 minutes.

Happy Relationships

Of course, it goes without saying that all of us have mastered the finer art of balanced relationships. If only it were true.

Dr. John Gray, author of the tremendously successful book, "Men are from Mars, Women are from Venus", seems to have hit the nail on the head when it comes to describing how men and women interact with each other.

Dr. Gray points out that men and women have fundamentally different needs and it is through recognizing what these needs are and appreciating the differences, that understanding and harmony blossoms.

A happy relationship is one where each person understands that it is not their job to make the other happy. Instead, they work on becoming the best person they can be and then share themselves deeply, openly and intimately without hesitation.

Getting to know someone is a lifetime pursuit. We never truly get to know anyone a hundred percent because even we don't know ourselves this much.

That's why the happiest relationships are those that never take each other for granted and are always looking to keep the relationship fresh, spontaneous, and alive by valuing it enough to want to put in an effort each day to make it fun and adventurous.

HERE'S HOW TO SPEND THE NEXT 5 MINUTES

Make a list of as many things as you can think of that are fun and new that you can do with your partner. Then, starting today, do something different with them every day. Really let your imagination go to town here as you partner is most definitely worth it.

These don't have to be massive events either. It can be as simple as greeting them at the door and giving them a big hug and kiss as soon as they get home and telling them how wonderful it is to see them. It's not about what you do together, it's about how genuine your intent is to connect with them and show them that they are loved.

Mirroring - Reflections of You

When you take the time to gaze closely into a mirror what do you see? Do you peruse yourself lovingly, without any criticism? Or does a frown appear upon your forehead as you ponder the ways in which you can create a more appealing image?

What you see reflected in the mirror is how you view the world around you. Either you are open and allowing, or you are critical and rigid. Other people are mirrors to your inner world. They offer you the opportunity to gaze into your sub-conscious mind and beliefs, and identify whether you are accepting or rejecting parts of your being.

Think about those people you enjoy being with. What are they reflecting back to you about yourself? They reveal those aspects of your ego personality that you are comfortable and happy with. On the other hand, the people you do not enjoy being with, reveal those aspects of your ego that you are critical of.

As we mature and get more comfortable with who we are as a whole person, it gets easier to be more accepting of a wider variety of reflections that people show to us.

Did you know that the greatest growth in relationships generally comes from those whom you are most challenged by? If this surprises you then think back to all the times that you have avoided, side-stepped, rejected or fled from situations that were unpleasant or challenging.

One thing for sure is that whatever reflection you run away from will almost always come back to haunt you. It may have a different name, face, or identity, yet at the same time there will be an eerie feeling of déjà vu.

Judgment Day

Until you have released the need to be judgmental you will always have it reflected back to you in your relationships. A safe and comfortable relationship often means a controlled one. This behavior exemplifies the lack of personal power that is created when you allow yourself to be manipulated through fear.

The fear for a person who controls others is that if there is no one to control then they do not feel powerful. The fear for a person who is controlled is that without someone to control them they feel powerless to create their own life.

The first step in releasing the need to either control or be controlled is to become aware of which pattern is most obvious for you. Sometimes both will be true but one trait will always be slightly more dominant than the other.

Allowing yourself to be treated like a doormat builds resentment and unhappiness. Traditionally, it is the male who has always portrayed the dominant role while the female played out the opposite. These days the tides have turned to some extent, although not quite as far as it can.

Women are now looking for more in themselves and their partners than playing second fiddle. Both men and women need to learn how to live in balance within themselves and together. This is already starting to gather momentum around the world yet there is still a long way to go.

Frequently, when coaching people having relationship challenges I hear such statements as:

- *'He did....!'*
- *'She did.....!'*
- *'"They did....!'*
- *'What did I do to deserve this?'*
- *'Why is this happening to me?"*

In reply to these statements I will say to them:

- *'How did you FEEL about this?'*
- *'How did you FEEL about that?'*
- *'What are you FEELING right now?'*

Notice how the first sentences focus on blame and victimization whereas the latter enables you to:

- Release blame.
- Retain your power.
- Take full responsibility for your experiences.
- Resolve your inner conflict.

Another important clue to releasing victimhood comes from asking yourself, "What can I learn about myself from this experience, and how can this knowledge assist me to choose more happiness in my life?"

The idea is to catch your thoughts and feelings before they overwhelm you and become a rampaging monster. Once the monster is loose it can be exhausting trying to put it back in its cage. Catch your thoughts and feelings as they happen then there is no monster to take care of.

The good news is that the more you practice this technique, the easier it gets. I have discovered that focusing on a negative emotion for more than one minute is indulgence. One minute is all you need to catch the feeling, focus on it, create change, and choose how you want to deal with it.

Right now, some of you may be sitting, or lying down with your mouth gaping open in disbelief. I understand, I used to be addicted to my dramas as well. It's okay to spend minutes, hours, days, or even years feeling sorry for yourself or angry at life but what use is it really?

Does it make your life any easier? Do your relationships improve? Are you any better off? Are you energized? Is it a pleasurable experience?

These are good questions to ask yourself when you get stuck in negativity. Only your mind gets stuck because it judges negative emotions as being unpleasant. The solution of course is to begin a new mental diet. If your mind can be conditioned to judge your negative thoughts and feelings, you can certainly train it to respond to them in a positive and constructive way.

Only you can tell your mind where to focus, how to focus and on what to focus. This can be done in a moment. It is as simple as taking several slow, deep breaths, or choosing to focus on solutions, rather than problems. In either case, immediate change can be created, providing instant relief from potentially overwhelming situations.

The fastest way to let go of a judgmental mind
is to stop judging that you judge.
Then, the next step is simple.

Mental and Emotional Mastery

To master your mind and emotions is to master your life. Especially when you think about how crazy life is for so many people and what they do just to cope that shows how little control they have over these areas.

Too many of us leave ourselves at the mercy of outside events, which we tend to have little or no control over and fail to take charge of our mind or emotions – which we can control – and rely instead on things like alcohol, cigarettes, drugs, anti-depressants and all sorts of harmful quick fixes.

We know inside ourselves that applying these quick fixes is not going to solve anything for us long-term. But because some of the emotions we experience are so intense and we are conditioned to avoid them at all costs, we look for the easiest way to cope so we don't come unstuck.

Really, there is no thought or emotion that is more powerful than you and your freedom to choose who you want to be. All you need is a simple way to take back your power from your conditioned reactive behaviors and step into a more enlightened way of being.

I call this self mastery.

To have mastery, or control as it can also be called, over your mind and emotions is to have control over your life – nothing else is needed.

Taking control of your life begins with creating space in your head. When you have space to think and act in a way that is more assertive, rather than reactive, then you are on the path to a happier, healthier, and more productive life.

There are some really simple tools that I have learned to help create more space for you to take control of your thoughts and feelings. The best time to apply these is as soon as you notice that you are having negative thoughts or feelings.

These tools include:

- Taking several, slow, deep breaths before you make a decision or take any action.
- Focusing on solutions to challenges, rather than get stuck on the problems.
- Ask empowering questions of yourself like:
  o What can I learn from this?
  o How can I make this better?
  o What am I feeling?

- Do something physical (i.e. running, swimming, dancing, gym, yoga, tai-chi, etc).
- Write your thoughts down in a journal.
- Walk away from the situation and come back to it when you are calmer.
- Give yourself some physical space.
- Do an active meditation to help release your emotions and calm your mind.

These are just a few of the ways to help yourself rapidly shift any negative emotions you may be experiencing. Always keep in mind that what works for someone else may not necessarily work for you. You may need to try a few different things before you find the best method for you.

HERE'S HOW TO SPEND THE NEXT 5 MINUTES

Have a blank page in front of you and for the next five minutes write down whatever comes into your head. Don't judge or censor it in any way – just let your words be whatever they are.

Just observe your thoughts and write what you see. If any feelings arise while you do this just keep on writing and let your emotions flow into your words. Then, as soon as you notice that you are feeling calm again, stop writing, close your eyes, and just relax for a few moments.

The Neutral Zone

Sometimes, the only peace and calmness that people have in their relationships are those rare moments between battles. The love that once existed becomes a memory buried deep beneath the remnant of a war-torn environment.

There are often many wounds to be healed in these relationships. This healing can only happen if you are both willing to make love and happiness more important than war.

Don't wait for things to get out of hand before you realize that the spark between you is now a place of numbness or despair. It always takes two to tango, so if you are caught in a battle zone then ask yourself what you are getting out of the fight.

No behavior is without compensation even if it is unpleasant. If you are addicted to conflict this will be evident by the battlefield you find yourself participating in.

Rekindling the Fire

One of the questions I always get asked is "How do you keep the spark alive once the honeymoon is over in a relationship?" Ask yourself this question. Why are you with your partner? Is it for any of the following reasons?

- Security
- Safety
- Comfort
- Habit
- Fear of being alone
- Sacrifice (for the children's sake)

If so then it's no surprise that your relationship may feel like it's too much hard work.

Do you remember the first time you met your partner or fell head over heels in love with someone? Do you remember the excitement, the passion, the desire, and the butterflies in the stomach that came with this love? Are these qualities a part of your relationships now?

These experiences are more powerful when you first meet someone because of the "thrill of the chase." Once the chase is over, you are then faced with 'managing' the relationship. This is when the love affair can be allowed to become routine and mundane, or taken for granted as it is called.

The time honored tradition of marriage gives us interesting insights into the functions and dysfunctions of couples. The Bureau of Statistics tells us that at least fifty percent of married couples will either separate or divorce.

This indicates that at least half of all people who get married have no idea how to manage a long-term relationship with someone who has different ways of thinking and behaving to theirs.

There are not many issues that can't be resolved through effective communication and the willingness to let love and happiness be more important than anything that may be driving a wedge between you.

When relationships enter the 'managing' phase certain symptoms can start to appear such as:

- Too tired to make love
- Not listening to your partner
- Uninterested in sharing experiences
- Spending more time apart from each other
- Seeking attention outside the relationship
- Irritability within the other person
- Depression and anxiety
- Boredom and complacency

If you are married, living with or involved with someone in a long-term commitment then the chances are that you have come across some of these symptoms yourself.

For your relationship to move beyond feeling like you are doing more than treading water with no land in site, there are a few important steps that you can take.

Firstly, ask yourself, "Do I want to stay in this relationship?" Then be honest about the answer, without letting sentiment or fear sway your judgment. If the answer is "yes" then you can take the next step. If the answer is "no", then what are you willing to do about it?

Rekindling the fire within a relationship that has lost its spark will take diligent effort at first. You have to be willing to commit time, energy, and effort to generate enough heat to fuel the fire.

If you are not prepared to consciously work towards this goal then ask yourself what is motivating you to stay in the relationship. Secondly, ask yourself, "Am I staying in this relationship out of love, or fear?"

From love it looks like, "I am willing to commit to creating the highest experience of happiness and joy possible with every breath I take, both within myself and my relationship."

From fear it looks like, "I am willing to put up with misery and pain because that is all I am worthy of receiving in my life."

If your answer is love, then every morning upon awakening, ask yourself what you and your partner can explore about each other on this day that you have not explored before.

This will bring newness back into everything you do together. Adopting an attitude of newness is a simple technique to instantly re-ignite passion in your relationship. All it takes is imagination and willingness to do it.

Once you get started it will blossom into a playful and creative way to share time and energy with your partner. While practicing newness allow yourself to be spontaneous and unusual, different, and daring. Let your imagination run free and see where it takes you.

One day, a student of Zen went to see his teacher. The student asked, *"What can I do? I feel like I am not getting anywhere with my spiritual practices."*

The Zen master replied, *"Go into the back yard and chase a chicken."*

"What shall I do with it when I catch it?" asked the puzzled student.

"I did not ask you to catch it, just chase it", replied the teacher.

We have become so goal oriented that we have forgotten the simple pleasure of enjoying where we are and what we have. There is an abundance of inspiration within every moment, if only you take the time to look.

If you focus too intensely on where you are going, rather than where you are, you may stumble and fall into some unseen pothole. Make each step you take the most important one, then you will enjoy a smoother ride.

Want Versus Need

Another point that is worth mentioning is the difference between *want* in a relationship and *need*. If you are in a relationship for any reason other than the joy of it then perhaps it is conditional upon a need.

To be with someone out of need is a love based on fear. When a relationship is founded upon fear the possibility of destructive traits such as revenge, possessiveness and jealousy emerging is highly likely.

These things bring out the ugliness and potential violence within people and do nothing except create more pain and suffering in people's lives. If your relationship is based on this behavior, be thankful that you are reading this now so you can choose what you really want your love life to look like.

'Want' is when you choose to be in a relationship to heighten the experience of happiness and joy that you already have in your life. If you need someone in your life to be happy, then you have not yet learned that true happiness comes from within.

A happy and healthy relationship does not include neediness. The energy of neediness is one of taking, rather than giving because the person who is needy has something missing inside them and they want you to fill in that space.

The problem arises when you decide you don't want to be the one to fill that need all the time. Then all hell can break loose and you then become the reason that they are in pain.

Can you see how this is a no-win situation? That's why it's better to not give in to a needy person – ever. Because the moment you fill their needs, then they will expect you to be there – all the time. And, unless you are a saint, eventually you will grow tired of it, and resent having to fulfill someone else's emotional needs.

We all have emotional baggage from the past that we need to deal with and sometimes we can work this out with another person, and sometimes we can't. The point is to know the difference between when you are working together with someone to grow beyond your own limitations in a mutually responsible way, or it's a struggle to find a common meeting ground where both parties fell fulfilled.

Treat others the way you want to be treated and you will attract the most amazing people into your life.

There are no accidents when it comes to whom you attract into your life. You will always have the exact person you need for where you are at. That's why if you don't get the lesson that they came to teach you, then you'll find the exact same person knocking on your door with a different name and face, but the same lessons to be learned.

By treating others how you want to be treated you will break free from your past and break through to relationships that make your heart sing and your life together a joy.

Affirmations

These are handy and powerful tools to magnetize into your life what you truly want and desire. You already understand that all life is energy, so it makes sense that what you focus on most of the time is eventually what you will get back in life.

If you run around all day affirming how bad your relationships are or how you always attract the wrong people into your life, then this will become a self fulfilling prophecy.

Fortunately, there are ways to focus your energy so that you can harness its positive potential whenever you like. That's what an affirmation does.

An affirmation is a process of thought training. They are the easiest and simplest techniques you can use to affect the conscious mind. An affirmation is a statement that you continuously repeat to yourself silently or aloud, depending on what suits you best at the time.

You can do affirmations anywhere – waiting at the doctor's office, driving your car, standing in a queue, while having a shower, or lying in your bed before going to sleep. The best part is that you get to decide upon the statement you want to use that best represents what you really want to have, be, or do.

It is recommended to always affirm what you want in the present tense. The reason for this is that your brain doesn't know the difference between what is real or what is imagined. It only knows what you tell it.

For example, if you are worried about something, then you mind is currently focused on something that is

142

obviously causing tension. Let's say you want to feel calm and relaxed instead, then you could use an affirmation like, "As I breathe in I feel relaxed and as I breathe out I am calm." This is quietly repeated to yourself for up to 5-minutes.

The technique above is a more mindful way to do affirmations as it is connecting an affirmation to your breath in and your breath out. It's not always important to do this but if you're looking to make changes in the way you feel then this is a very powerful tool.

Normally, with affirmations though you can simply repeat a statement in your mind such as, "I am relaxed, and calm", as a way to influence the thoughts in your mind. Your mind can only handle one thought at a time so the power of affirmations comes from filling your mind with thoughts that reinforce what you want to happen to you.

Think of it this way. Everything that you currently experience in your life from your health and happiness, to the car you drive, the friends you have and the work you do, have all come from the thoughts you have given power to, the majority of the time.

That's why people who are constantly suffering from excessive fear, stress, or worry sometimes find it so hard to be free from them because the mind gets stuck on negative thought patterns that help to keep reproducing the same result in their lives.

Affirmations do not necessarily lead to instant change. The power for them to transform your life comes from constant repetition over time. That's why using an affirmation for just 5-minutes a day, every day, is one of the smartest investments you could make in yourself and your future life.

You don't have to believe what you are affirming. Instead, just keep repeating it as your sub-conscious mind is listening.

That's why an affirmation can be so powerful. The constant repetition of an affirmation assists in transforming the energy of past belief systems that are blocking the object of your desire from becoming a reality.

If you persevere, eventually any limiting and self-sabotaging beliefs will be replaced by the new, improved, life-giving affirmations. A self-sabotaging belief may look like, 'I am not worthy of being loved', which results in people coming into your life that use you rather than love you.

People who dislike their bodies or judge themselves to be unattractive can have this belief system. It can lead to fear of intimacy, sexual repression, aloofness, or even low self-esteem. To change this belief system, you could use an affirmation such as 'I am worthy to give and receive love in every moment.'

At first, you may not believe what you are telling yourself. If you keep reinforcing your new belief on a daily basis and empower it with actions that are aligned with your desired goal, then your affirmation will soon become a part of your daily experiences.

Sometimes, you may fall back into your old habits. If this happens, instead of being disillusioned, acknowledge the changes you have achieved and keep reinforcing your new belief, until it is fully integrated.

In the above example you could start by allowing your needs to be met. If you need to be hugged, ask for a hug instead of moping around feeling sorry for yourself. If you don't feel like doing the dishes after dinner, then give yourself permission to make this choice, without worrying about what others think or say.

There are infinite ways to show yourself and those around you that you are ready, willing, and able to transform your life and achieve your goals. Always be prepared to declare to life what you want and follow through with appropriate action to reinforce your declaration.

Another important point to consider is to let go of a time frame regarding 'when' the affirmation is going to work for you. The fact is that as soon as you affirm anything, be it positive, or negative, it has already happened energetically. It just takes time for it to take shape in the physical world.

When you start using affirmations, be sure that you are ready to receive what you are asking for. If you are not ready, then like a ship sailing by on a foggy night, your opportunities may come and go unnoticed, like they have many times before.

HERE'S HOW TO SPEND THE NEXT 5 MINUTES

Pick an area of your life that you want to change. Write down an affirmation that fits in with your desired outcome. Let's say you want to feel more happiness in your life; then you could use an affirmation like, "I love life and life loves me". Then repeat it silently or aloud to yourself right now for the next few minutes.

Remember that you can use your affirmations throughout your day to help accomplish the things you want. They are easy to say and can be done anywhere and what's even better is that you don't have to even believe them – just repeat them!

Visualizations

Visualizations can be used in conjunction with affirmations or on their own as a powerful medium for attracting what you want. Visualizations are about using your imagination to see yourself in a situation that hasn't happened yet, picturing having or doing the thing you want and successfully achieving your desired outcome.

For example, let's say you want to be more productive with your time and energy. Using visualization you picture yourself as being productive. You see yourself doing things, getting through tasks and achieving your goals, all with ease, calmness, and with plenty of time to spare.

Visualization is a powerful tool because everything that exists in the physical world came from someone's imagination.

Look around you at all the products and services that began with someone's idea that we now take for granted such as toilet paper and television. Two hundred years ago, no one dreamed of space travel yet with imagination we are now entering an era of deep space exploration. So to say that our imagination is powerful is an understatement. It's the most powerful mind tool that we have at our disposal yet all too many leave it to its own devices, rather than try to harness its power.

Visualizations offer you a convenient, entertaining, and effective way to get what you want. The best way to harness their power is to:

1. Choose what you want to be, do, or have: lose weight, gain confidence, start a business, fall in love, travel overseas, et cetera.
2. Take a few minutes to relax your body and mind. If you can, try doing a simple meditation technique for before you start visualizing. It will help put you into an optimal state. If not, just sit or lie down and relax.
3. Spend five to ten minutes visualizing the reality you want.
4. Most importantly, always visualize in the present tense. This means that you are imagining something that's important to you as if it's already happening to you right now.

The images that you create in your head are like mini-movies that you get to focus the power of your mind and thoughts on in a repetitious manner. You need to visualize what you want daily for weeks or months until your goal has been achieved. Any thought that you put into your mind and focus on regularly will produce results.

Don't worry about getting the picture perfect as some people don't see images in their head so easily. Instead, you might want to make yourself a vision board of what you want and then gaze at it for a few minutes a day and let it sink into your sub-conscious mind through your eyes.

It also helps to add detail to your visualizations. Pretend you are watching a motion picture in your head, only this time it is fully interactive, and you are the star, director, and producer. You can use everything that you see in the movies: color, contrast, scenery, objects, sound, music, emotions, smell, taste, touch, and any sensation you can think of.

For example, let's say you desire a partner to share your life with. Then be as detailed as possible about what you are asking for.

- What does this person look like?
- What color is their hair?
- What sort of personality do they have?
- Where do they work?
- How tall are they?
- How does their skin feel when you touch it?
- What fragrances do they wear?
- How does their voice sound?
- What are their interests?
- What do you feel in your heart?

Don't be concerned about how things will unfold and in what timeframe. These things can't be controlled. Instead, trust the process and know that your mind is the most powerful tool you have at your disposal to change your life. All change begins in your mind.

Sometimes you will attract something other than what you thought you wanted but nonetheless it turns out to be perfect for you. Life knows what we really want and need, more so than we do ourselves at times. Sometimes we can become so anxious to achieve a goal that we become fixated on a rigid idea rather than remembering to go with the flow of life and the blessings that are already being given to us – even if we don't see them straight away.

Just by visualizing what you want to have, be, or do on a regular basis, situations and opportunities will come your way that will lead you to your goal – of this you can be sure.

Above all, have fun with your affirmations and visualizations and know that at the very least you will spend some time each day focusing on positive energy, rather than limitations or negativity.

HERE'S HOW TO SPEND THE NEXT 5 MINUTES

Decide on something you want to be, do, or have. Then close your eyes and start picturing it in your mind as if you already have achieved it. Fill in as much detail as you can and allow yourself to feel the feelings of what it is like to have achieved your goal. If it makes you feel happy, then let your body be filled with happiness as you visualize your desired outcome. Feel yourself smiling and see yourself smiling in your mini-movie. The more positive feelings you can add to your visualization, the more powerful it will be.

Follow this process for anything you want to have, become or do in your life for five minutes a day.

Mind Power

Many years ago I worked as an assistant for an organization called Mind Powers. One night, one of the instructors shared with us a few of his goals. They were:

- *To be married within six months*
- *To double his current salary working less hours*
- *To have a new house and car within one month*

David informed us that he was using affirmations and visualizations every day in the morning before getting out of bed and at night as he fell asleep.

Two weeks later David gathered us all together again and informed us that he had already met the woman of his dreams, had been offered a new job that was less hours and higher pay and he could now afford a bigger house and pay off a new car.

A few months later we were all invited to David's wedding at his new house. If I had any doubts as to the power of thought, emotion, and passion to create new realities, they ended with David's inspirational triumph over conditioned beliefs

The only thing that prevents you getting what you really want is what your subconscious clings to as its primary beliefs. These can be changed at any moment. If you doubt it, have a go for yourself and watch what happens.

Here's a list of qualities that are encouraged to be focused on in all relationships.

Powerful Relationships Are:

- WONDERFUL
- CREATIVE
- GROWTHFUL
- EMPOWERING
- CONNECTED
- PEACEFUL
- SENSATIONAL
- FUN
- ETERNAL
- TIMELESS
- EMBRACING
- MYSTERIOUS
- DIVINE

- ADVENTUROUS
- ENJOYABLE
- CARING
- LASTING
- SHARING
- FLEXIBLE
- FREE
- PERFECT
- ENLIGHTENING
- SIMPLE
- WHOLESOME
- AWESOME
- PLEASURABLE

The key to a lasting and fulfilling relationship is to be alive within it. Aliveness thrives on happiness and vitality. This does not necessarily mean that you will never have a disagreement. It means that you will deal with conflict in a more responsible manner.

Use these opportunities to strengthen your confidence and self esteem to easily deal with any future crisis, or cut them off at the bud before they begin. Either way you can sit back and enjoy the fruits of your labor.

Enjoy all your relationships especially the ones you find challenging as they are your opportunity to grow.

Appreciate everything and everyone in your life while you can because nothing lasts forever and whatever energy you give out to those around you is exactly what you will get back.

To assist in having healthy, happy, and vibrant relationships choose one of the affirmations in the table below each day and not only affirm it but live it.

Pretty soon you will find that you have so many new friends who want to be with you, that you will forget any difficulties you may have had relating to people.

Affirmations for Love

♥ *I now deserve love, happiness, and peace in every moment of my life.*

♥ *I love my life and my life is simple and joyful.*

♥ *My partner and I enjoy increasing happiness and love.*

♥ *I have a joyous and intimate relationship with someone who loves me for who I am.*

♥ *Each day I am allowing more, and more love, into my life.*

♥ *I am willing to give freely and expect nothing in return.*

♥ *I am fulfilled by the joy of giving.*

♥ *I love that I live and I allow more love each day.*

♥ *I am always safe in my relationships, and love comes easily and effortlessly.*

♥ *My partner and I enjoy great sex.*

♥ *I always attract greatness into my life.*

♥ *I am at peace with my existence.*

♥ *My heart is open to give and receive love - equally.*

♥ *I forgive myself for holding on to the past when all I ever wanted was love.*

♥ *All my relationships are loving and harmonious.*

FIRST CLASS FLYING

Where Your Attitude Determines Your Altitude

"I'm sorry sir; the flight is full!" the reservations officer apologetically exclaimed.

These are the least cherished words that a stand-by passenger likes to hear while waiting to get a seat on the next plane out. Stand-by tickets are the ones you buy at the airline counter to save time and money; at least that is how it usually works.

The airport terminal was packed with weary travelers. Most were sporting newly acquired clothing and different degrees of overcooked skin. The last time I had seen this many people in one place was in New York City during peak hour traffic.

Compassionately, I thanked the airline officer for his time and asked if I could be placed on a list in case any seats became available. Then, I again thanked him for his assistance and complimented him on the way he was handling the onslaught of grumbling holiday makers.

The officer smiled for a moment in gratitude and said, "I'm glad someone noticed that I am doing my best given the circumstances."

It felt good to have lightened this man's day, even if only for a moment.

As I walked away from the counter it struck me that I was now officially stuck at Bali's Denpasar International Airport.

There were many of us waiting to see if we could get on this flight. I watched several frustrated people approach the counter and demand special attention for reasons I'm sure even they didn't believe.

I wondered how many people could have a dying relative at home, a pregnant wife in the wings or a sudden medical condition that happened on the last day of their holiday.

I realized that I had placed myself in an interesting predicament. I was due back at work by 9.00am tomorrow morning. Yesterday, my wallet had been stolen from my hotel room; and today the airline staff informed me that all flights home were completely filled for the next month.

Broke, stranded and with no backup plan, I decided to forget about my plight and do something relaxing. Searching through my baggage I came across my favorite Eric Van Lustbader paperback novel and sat down to enjoy the adventures of Nicholas Linnear in 'The Ninja'.

I became so engrossed in the story that I completely forgot about going home until the reservations officer came rushing towards me and gasping for breath exclaimed, "Come quickly, the plane is about to depart and I think I may have found a seat for you!"

I quickly gathered my things and followed the officer to the counter. Without a word he took my bag, checked it in, issued me a boarding pass with seat "1A" typed in bold letters on it and wished me a pleasant flight home. I looked at my boarding pass in amazement.

"This is first class", I exclaimed in surprise.

"Yes", replied the officer with a grin, "We had someone no-show for the flight and this is the seat they were booked in. I do hope you enjoy your trip home."

I was the only stand-by passenger to get on the flight that day. I was aware that many had put their name down before me and I also realized that a simple comment of appreciation had gone a lot further than a mouthful of complaining.

But choosing to stay calm and relaxed and be okay with what was happening instead of trying to fight it, everything ended up working out in way I could not have imagined.

The future is never predestined. Every page in the book of your life is blank until you fill them with the choices you make. If the choices you make flow from appreciation, then your future will always be appreciated.

What on Earth is Self-Worth?

Self-worth is your positive or negative evaluation of the self in relationship to psychological well being. It also means the experience of being competent to cope with the basic challenges of life, and being worthy of happiness and given respect.

You are already a worthy being. All that is needed is your acceptance of it.

Our self-worth is derived from many factors that have shaped the way we view ourselves. The interesting thing is that we can have high self worth in some areas while being low in others. For example, some people can be very strong in their roles at work and be authoritative and handle problems competently, while in personal relationships they give their power away.

What creates the difference? Your internal beliefs about how you view yourself in the differing roles or identities that you enact in life. Some people may have a strong self-image when it comes to making money yet have a low self-image when it comes to how their body looks. This would result in them being good at making money and putting on weight easily or getting sick frequently.

Self-worth is one of the most important areas of our lives to work on improving. Any area of your life where you feel weak or disempowered will be coming from a lack of self worth. The great news about this is that you can work at increasing your self-worth quite quickly and easily.

My friend Mary had been going through a tough relationship breakup and decided to relocate to a new city and have a fresh start. So she packed up her belongings and shifted across the country.

Within two weeks of arriving at her new place Mary landed a job with a prominent real estate firm. During the first week Mary was asked to take on an assignment that everyone else in the office said couldn't be done.

Mary's task was to sell a large section of undeveloped land that was subdivided, had several owners, and was poorly located according to current market trends. None of the agents had been able to sell any of the blocks in over a year, so they had all given up trying.

Mary had an idea that she wanted to test. Her idea was to approach the owners individually and asked each of them if they were willing to be creative with their sales. At first, only one owner said yes.

Two days later, Mary approached the owner with a deal that consisted of swapping rental properties plus some residual cash in exchange for his land. The deal went ahead.

The owner was ecstatic, the buyer was happy and Mary pocketed a tidy sum from two commissions. By the end of her first month, Mary had successfully sold all the 'problem' blocks earning herself a tidy commission and a great deal of respect from her peers and clients.

The only time your self-worth is in question is when you doubt it. Forget about what others think you are capable of doing or not doing. That is just their opinion. When you stop comparing yourself with others and don't put unrealistic expectations on what you can and can't do then your self-worth will grow in leaps and bounds.

Self-worth also expands when you overcome challenges. The more you prove to yourself that you can rise above your challenges the easier it will be to resolve future challenges. There will never really be a time that you are not challenged in some way or another. However, there will come a time that you handle everything that comes your way with strength of character and confidence in your ability to get through it.

Keep telling yourself that you love and approve of yourself no matter what is going on in your life. Through good and bad times keep affirming this truth because one day you will believe it, and when you do, nothing will ever again be able to take away your happiness or peace.

HERE'S HOW TO SPEND THE NEXT 5 MINUTES

Pick an area of your life that you believe that you could improve your self-worth. Next, write down what it is you are afraid of. Next, close your eyes and visualize yourself as a super-confident person who can handle anything with ease.

To help with this think back to a time when you did feel confident and notice how your voice sounded and what your body language was. Then apply these feelings, sounds, and body postures to your new vision. You can also add-in an affirmation, if you like, to reinforce the entire process.

Risky Business

Living in fear is no fun. Another way to overcome your fears is to step outside your comfort zones. Take the chance to discover that your fears are only imagined. Taking a risk does not mean causing harm to yourself. It means challenging yourself to do things differently so you can improve one or many areas of your life.

For example, when I made the transition from having a job to working for myself I had to take a risk. The risk was to let go of the security of getting a weekly paycheck that sustained my lifestyle. Yes, it was scary and yes, it wasn't easy as those who have taken this leap of faith will know.

I had no idea if my business was going to work when I first started out but what I did have was enough self-worth to know that I had to give it my best shot or spend the rest of my life feeling like I'd cheated myself out of doing something real with my life.

It's better to regret the things you've done, than regret the things you haven't done.

Taking risks is essential to growth. As the saying goes, 'nothing ventured, nothing gained', and this is so very true when it comes to living your full potential. When you do the same things you've always done you'll always end up with the same or similar results. To have, be, or do more than what you have in the past you need to do things differently to create a better future.

If you are not sure what those things are that you need to do differently, then ask someone or put yourself in a position to find out. There will be a book, a video or a coach somewhere that will help you get off the treadmill of drudgery you may be stuck on. The key is to take some or any action that'll start moving your life in a new and exciting direction.

The Winning Streak

Look at your right hand for a moment. Now lift it up over your left shoulder and pat yourself on the back a few times. How often do you give yourself a reward for what you have achieved or even just for being who you are? Positive reinforcement is a great way to remind yourself that you are doing a good job.

Spend more time acknowledging what you do achieve regardless of how small or insignificant it may appear to be. At the same time give less energy towards your failures. Notice them like you would a cloud in the sky. Be detached from them and watch them float by until they have vanished over the horizon.

Telling yourself that you are a wonderful person is an important step forward in releasing what you believe is wrong with you. Spend less time worrying about what other people think of you and more time developing your personal power.

If you keep waiting for others to tell you how wonderful you are you may be in for a very long wait. The more you believe in yourself, the more the world will look upon you and see the sparkle in your eyes, hear the laughter in your voice and feel the love of self you have emanating from your heart.

Many of us have been taught that being self-involved is selfish or arrogant. Now we have the chance to turn the other cheek and learn that we have to first be self-involved before we can be truly selfless and giving to others.

As soon as you are happy within yourself you will have true happiness to give to the world around you. Otherwise, your emotional tanks will become easily depleted and your energy levels will fade quickly. The fact is that if you do not give yourself the happiness, love, and respect that you deserve, then who will?

You were born a winner because you beat the odds when that single sperm that became you, beat a million others to fertilize the egg in your mother's womb. You started out a winner because that's what life intended. The only difference between now and then is that you may have forgotten that you always have been and always will be a winner in life.

The only time you can lose is when you give up on something that matters. If you never do that, then you can never lose. If there is something that you have given up on that you know is important to your happiness and fulfillment, then it's time to get back on the horse. Start riding again and don't stop until you have achieved the result you want.

HERE'S HOW TO SPEND THE NEXT 5 MINUTES

Write down as many things that you can think about that you have succeeded in. Really think outside the box about the hundreds of ways that you have already proven to yourself you are a success. Like when you successfully got out of bed this morning, or you successfully beat one million other sperm to fertilize the egg in your mother's womb that became you.

We are always succeeding at something but all too often we forget to acknowledge it. The more you see yourself as a success, the more success you will have and the easier it will be to achieve anything you want in life.

Amazing Grace

There are no mistakes, only experiences. It is only when you view life through colored glasses that your journey is less than perfect. Think back upon those times when you did achieve something that you didn't believe possible. How did you feel?

Every experience is worthwhile - if you don't judge it.

I know that when I overcome any obstacle a part of me is changed forever. At these times I discover new and exciting frontiers to explore, that I might not have found if circumstances were different.

When I first began personal development I was so keen to learn more, that common sense often went out the window. I remember attending a two week meditation course in America. At that time I was working full time for another company and had to use up the rest of my annual leave to do the course.

After having been back at work for only one month, I found out that there was a seven-day follow up course being held in two weeks time. I desperately wanted to go. Yet reasoning said that it was not possible. I had no leave to take, it was an extremely busy time of year work wise and two of our office staff were already going to be absent during that time.

I was determined to find a way to go. The first thing I did was to approach Tony, my boss, and ask for leave without pay. He listened attentively until I had finished before politely rejecting my request.

He pointed out all the reasons why it was impossible for me to have a week off before I added, "I am sure there is a way that both you and I can get what we want. Let's look at other options".

Tony said the only way he could see that I could have the week off was if everyone else worked overtime and pitched in to do my work. This was all I needed. I mustered up my courage and spoke with everyone in my section about my plans and asked them if they were willing to cover for me while I went overseas again.

Even I was surprised when every single person agreed to help out. Tears of gratitude welled in my eyes as I felt the love and support that my fellow teammates had displayed.

I then went back and showed Tony a makeshift roster that we had drawn up that detailed how and what everyone would do in order to balance the workload.

He seemed to be genuinely impressed by the amount of work that I had put into making this choice easier for both of us.

This experience offered me many lessons. I learned to stay focused on what I wanted until every possibility was exhausted. I learned the value of friendship. I learned the value of truthful expression. I learned the value of effective communication. I learned to stand by my decisions even if others thought I was crazy. Most of all I learned the value of teamwork.

This challenge made it easier for me to eventually be more daring in my life and start living the life of my dreams.

If you focus on obstacles as opportunities for growth, your life will evolve in leaps and bounds. Every time you overcome an obstacle you are rewarded with a realization of yourself that no amount of money, courses, therapies, or friends can give to you.

Never lose sight of what you want to achieve, regardless of how big or small your hurdles may appear to be. Growth from obstacles comes from how you handle them, not how well you can avoid them, or get others to take care of them for you.

Remain focused on your goals. Deal with each obstacle as if it is a blessing that has been sent to you from deep inside you to awaken your slumbering consciousness. If your heart is only allowed to feel the burdens of your life and not the lightness and joy of it, then one day it may be so barren that it breaks from pain.

Never Give Up

When I first left conventional employment and decided to only live what brought me joy, I came upon many hurdles. The first obstacle appeared when I attempted to organize my first ever 'personal growth' workshop and no one booked in.

Instead of being disheartened, I focused on changing my approach. The next time I promoted the same workshop, over fifty people attended. The only difference between the two was the quality of questions I asked myself. Instead of asking myself what did I do wrong? I asked myself the question 'how else could I promote my workshop'?

*If you ask better questions you will
get better answers.*

Questions have incredible power to shape thoughts and day-to-day experiences. To consistently produce the results you desire, this must be reflected in the type of questions you put out to the world.

Questions:

- *Why is this happening to me?*
- *What did I do to deserve this?*
- *Where did I go wrong?*

The questions only help you to focus on the problem, not look for a solution. The quickest and easiest way to change focus is to ask new and empowering questions.

Instead, ask questions like:

- *How can I improve my situation?*
- *What can I learn from this experience to become stronger?*
- *What are my options, even if I have to ask others for help?*

It won't matter as much what happens in your life if you are willing to focus on questions that turn desperation into inspiration.

Attitude of Gratitude

Just the other day I was counseling a course participant. As I sat there listening to her complain about what was wrong with her life, which mainly concerned her partner, I became aware that everything she was expressing was coming from criticism.

If you can release judgment for just one day you will be well on your way to a happier, healthier, and more productive life. You will discover that criticism, especially self-criticism, keeps you bound in misery.

By converting the focus of your energy from criticism to gratitude you will enhance your life and the lives of those you love. The more time and energy you spend on being negative the more of your life you waste.

On one occasion my friend Mark tried to pull a trick on me by telling me that the clothes I had on were in bad taste. Instead of getting defensive or upset about the comment, I replied with, "thank you, I take that as a compliment because I am a master of bad taste."

Mark looked at me in disbelief and then we both roared in laughter. Later on Mark shared with me that he had expected me to say something sarcastic back and was at a loss for words when I didn't.

If you want to experience the uplifting power of gratitude instead of the destructive power of criticism, then for one whole day from the moment you get up to the moment you fall asleep resolve to develop a winning attitude:

HERE'S HOW TO SPEND THE NEXT 5 MINUTES

Read out loud all the affirmations below. Notice which one connects with you the most and then focus on repeating it to yourself daily until it becomes part of your mindset.

- *I will criticize nothing that happens today.*
- *I will imagine that everything that happens is for my highest good.*
- *I will release myself from any judgments I have of myself.*
- *I will hold a vision of myself, my motivations, and my actions as pure.*
- *I will not agree with the critical words or attitudes of others.*
- *I will look for goodness within and around me.*
- *I will celebrate the entire day with an attitude of gratefulness towards everything that I give and receive.*

THE KEY TO SELF LOVE

The View from the Roof

Sarah was like a gift from God to me as she had a way of opening my heart like no one else could. Sarah lived in the body of a child, but her lessons taught to me were like from an ancient master. I learned to chase butterflies for the sake of chasing, dance for the sake of dancing, sing for the sake of singing, and play for the sake of playing.

Sarah would ask me questions about God such as, *"What is God like?"*

To which I would say, *"God is just like you."*

One Saturday afternoon I decided to visit Sarah and her family at their new house in the city. As soon as I arrived Sarah took me on a guided tour of the house. My first thoughts were how small the living space was and my heart went out to such a beautiful family living under such restrictive conditions.

Each room that Sarah entered came alive as she enthusiastically guided me through the small dwelling. As soon as we had finished the tour Sarah could hardly contain her excitement as she blurted out, *"Would you like to see my secret room?"*

"You bet", I replied enthusiastically.

Sarah took me by the hand and guided me out to the tiny back yard, where the side fence connected with the back wall. Then I watched with intrigue as she nimbly climbed the fence and sat waiting upon the first level of the roof. Without hesitation I followed.

Soon we were both lying on top of the roof watching the sun slowly sinking beneath the vastness of the inner city skyline. Sarah turned towards me with her face all lit up and exclaimed;

"This is my favorite room in the house. I always come up here and play with the birds and speak to people as they pass by. I love my roof."

I was stunned. I could see exactly what she meant. By creating this room, Sarah had opened up a whole new world to explore and enjoy. Amidst a concrete jungle of haste and limited space a small child had found a Garden of Eden where to most of us none could possibly exist.

Sarah's willingness to find life in all things put most spiritual people I knew to shame. I drove home in a state of awe. This thirteen-year-old saw her life through the eyes of innocence and appreciation, and that made all the difference.

It made me reconsider where I was lacking in gratitude for what I did have and how much time I spent focusing on what I didn't have. While focusing on limitations, I had overlooked the view from the roof. Now I too could find a roof, no matter where I went.

The Milk is Spilt - So What!

Have you ever noticed how some people appear to value things more than something that is alive? What if you broke your mother-in-law's favorite vase? How would you react? Would you feel guilt ridden or accept what you did and move on, not wasting a precious second dwelling on the past?

Accidents happen. We can't control everything that happens in our lives. Sometimes you will make mistakes and do stupid things. What really matters is how you deal with the unexpected when it happens.

If something like this were to happen so what! It doesn't have to be a big deal if you don't want it to be. Other people can and do choose to behave immaturely but you don't have to allow yourself to get pulled into their blame game unless you want to.

There is no reason in the world for you to ever be anything other than at peace with who you are. If you feel guilty about what happened, then deal with the feeling instead of giving your power away to others to control your life.

Anything that you place more value on than inner peace, harmony, and well-being will ultimately control the quality of your life.

You have only one main responsibility and that is to be true to yourself. Don't allow the attitudes, opinions or actions of others sway you from this path. If you try to take on the pain of the world, you will most likely drown in it.

No Time for Regrets

You are constantly allowing the expectations of others and the limits that you put on yourself to prevent you from exploring what your soul needs to journey in this lifetime. This is why so many people feel unfulfilled.

Who are you living for, if not for yourself? Don't wait until your body is aged and your mind is feeble before you finally admit to yourself that you didn't do half the things you really wanted to.

Regret will always follow compromise. By not compromising your hopes and dreams, and following your heart's desires you will have no time for regret.

If others get upset with your choices in life that's okay. It's really none of our business what others think or say about us. The more you can live this way, the less drama you'll end up attracting into your life.

Consider all those people who get upset by cyber trolls. It makes no sense to give faceless and nameless people so much power to control how we feel. It's all just a mind game that we play with ourselves. That's why it's so important to get to know who you really are because until you do, your state of mind and emotional wellbeing is not in your hands.

Living a life of no regrets means forgiving your past and learning how not to drag it into the future. From this moment on stop compromising your wants and needs just to keep the peace or make others happy. You are not responsible to make others happy – that is their job.

HERE'S HOW TO SPEND THE NEXT 5 MINUTES

Pick something you've been putting off doing that is important to you and take immediate action towards it. Even if it's just to write it down as a goal and put a date you want to achieve it by – it doesn't matter. What matters is that you start living your dreams and stop yourself from living a life of regret for the things you didn't say or do in your life – while you could.

INVALUABLE YOU

I Am Abundantly Happy

Let's take a look at one of the most misunderstood concepts of life and that is the one called abundance.

Firstly, let me define 'abundance' as:

To know, feel and enjoy the richness and fullness of every moment.

This means that if you are experiencing a moment filled with joy, then you are abundantly joyful; if you are experiencing a moment filled with sadness, then you are abundantly sad; if you are angry, then you have an abundance of anger.

In my experience there is an unlimited supply of everything that we will ever want or need in life. From money to motivation, health to happiness, or energy to creativity, it's all there for the taking. All you need to learn to do is to be open to receive it.

If every thought you think, word you speak, and action you take is focused on abundance then you can expect that you will instantly start to attract more abundance into your life. This is by far the simplest and quickest way to go from a life of lack to a life of plenty.

However, if you're always checking out your bank balance or recoiling in despair that things are not going well for you, then you can expect to attract even more to be desperate about. The reasoning for this is quite simple – what we put out energetically is what we get back and the two main energies we can focus on are either lack, or abundance.

Prosperous or Preposterous

There is such a vast opportunity for growth in this area that the question is not so much how can you become more abundant in your life. It's more how abundant and prosperous do you desire and deserve to be?

Without fail, if a person isn't doing well financially it's because they've bought into beliefs of lack. Prosperity of course is not just about money. It's so much bigger than that. It's about being rich in mind, body, spirit, and finances.

I view prosperity or prosperous thinking as the river that flows to the ocean of abundance that both surrounds us and lives within us. By building beliefs of prosperity into every area of your life and eliminating any beliefs of lack, you will not only change your circumstances but will also skyrocket your emotional fulfillment.

A financial survey recently revealed there is enough resources on the planet to evenly distribute at least one million dollars to every man, woman and child! These are interesting facts when you consider the unequal distribution of wealth that currently exists.

The wealthy play a numbers game in which actual dollars and cents are rarely seen. The dividends they receive through superior money management skills far exceed the almost worthless interest that the average person gains through local bank rates. The good news is that these skills can be learned.

Along with learning these skills you will also need a mindset of abundance. Without it, all the skills in the world won't matter as any money you do acquire will surely be lost.

To have financial wealth you must first release any addictions you may have to poverty. These addictions are found within your limiting belief systems regarding money. If you grew up in an environment where your parents constantly reinforced hardship, lack, and struggle then this is the first hurdle you need to navigate over.

The way to do that is to educate yourself on how financially independent people achieved this state of prosperity and then start doing what they did. Take baby steps if you need to, but just keep moving forward until your reach your desired financial destiny.

HERE'S HOW TO SPEND THE NEXT 5 MINUTES

Write down one area that you perceive any lack in your life. Then write down how it would look if it were abundant.

Now, close your eyes and imagine that you are five years in the future and you have carried this abundant part of you with you from now. Notice where you are, what you are doing, and how you feel having lived a life of abundance for the past five years. Let as many sounds, colors, and sensations of abundance wash over you as you can.

Then, come back to the present moment and take the memory of this experience and place it in your heart and say out loud, *"I am so happy with how abundant my life is in every way."*

Just a reminder that you can Grab this free guided meditation series to see how it works in practice.

www.MasterYourMindspace.com/meditationprogram

How Much Are You Worth?

Prosperity starts with you. If your passion is to be wealthy then spend time with people who have already achieved wealth. They will teach you more about building beliefs of prosperity than any amount of day-dreaming, hoping, or desiring will ever do.

What value do you currently place on your time? One of the ways to accurately measure this is to look at how much you currently value yourself in terms of financial reward.

This is worked out by adding up your sources of income and dividing them by the number of working hours in your day. This will give you an idea of how much one hour of your time is worth.

Let's say you earn $1,000.00 per week. If you work 40 hours for it then your current hourly rate is:

$1,000 divided by 40 hours = $25 per hour.

In this example your financial return for an hour of your working time is $25. This is what your current prosperity beliefs are generating as your financial worth.

Do you believe that you are worth more than your current financial return? Then set yourself a goal to double this rate over the next six months. I know it can be done because it happened for me.

Initially, I set myself a goal of doubling my income in half the amount of hours worked. This happened within six months. Since then I have learned that by supplying products or services to people that improve the quality of their life, and reaching the most amount of people possible in the shortest time brings great rewards to everyone. In short, I learned the power of leveraging my time and skills to maximize income.

This wisdom also applies to if you have a J.O.B. If you can develop new systems or strategies to decrease workload, improve productivity or generate new income for your company, what boss would not give you a raise, promotion or both?

Seven Keys to Financial Abundance

1. Enjoy whatever money and resources you already have. Being grateful for the cash flow or resources that you already have is one of the fastest ways to attract more into your life.

2. Learn new financial skills. Read books on wealth building, listen to audios from people who are

successful and attend seminars whenever you get the chance that will show you how to build multiple streams of income.

3. Seek out like-minded people to help you achieve your financial targets. Remember - *Teamwork makes the Dream work.*

4. Save at least 10% of all you earn. It may seem hard at first but set a budget, which includes putting aside savings and stick to it.

5. Invest your savings wisely. Use your savings to invest wisely to build long-term wealth and cash-flow. Having more than one source of income is essential to creating financial freedom. There are many ways to do this, from property to shares. Do what you love the most.

6. Have a written set of financial goals. Then work out some action steps you can take to make those goals happen. If your plan doesn't work, don't give up - make another plan. There is never anything wrong with any idea, there are only poor plans.

7. Take the work out of life and instead let life work for you. Your prosperity will naturally increase as you allow yourself to follow your heart and only do what brings you joy. If you don't know what you really want to do, then the first step is to discover what makes your heart sing.

Saving Face

Let's face it, very few people are good savers. This is largely due to a debt-based society and plenty of smart marketing gurus, peddling goodies to separate you from your hard earned dollars.

Imagine where you'd be financially if you had saved ten percent of your income from the very first dollar you ever earned. Makes you think doesn't it?

Saving is only one aspect of financial independence. The other is investing wisely. If you make the money you save grow for you, then your money is working for you.

It is quite true that a fool and their money are soon parted. So wise investing is the key. A general rule to follow for investing wisely is to only invest in people, products, or services that you have knowledge about.

If you are considering putting money into a project, always take the time to talk to those who have knowledge about it before making a decision, otherwise you may end up with burnt fingers.

The other point I'd like to make is that banks are a safe way to store funds, but not a good investment. By the time low interest rates, inflation, living expenses and fluctuations of the dollar eat away at your funds, you are usually no better off than sticking your money in an envelope under your bed.

Take the time to learn about wealth building. Study it, research it, and then find some area of wealth building that excites you and get started on your path to financial freedom.

A Matter of Worth

One day a friend of mine, Bob, was walking down the street when he noticed some money lying in the gutter. Bob bent down, picked up the loose bills, and to his astonishment realized that he was holding several hundred dollars.

Bob immediately assumed that someone nearby had lost it and eagerly looked around to find who it belonged to. The only other person he could see near him was a woman walking on the opposite side of the street.

Without hesitation he hurried across the street and breathlessly handed the woman the money as he blurted out, *"Excuse me, this must belong to you!"*

Then, feeling pleased with himself, Bob left without another word. At first, Bob felt relieved at having given away the money. Several minutes passed before Bob realized what he had just done. He had been so eager to give the money away, that he hadn't stopped to consider that it might not have belonged to the woman.

Have you ever given away money or rejected someone's offer of help because of guilt, fear, or pride. If you have, then this is something you'll need to change before you can become truly prosperous in every area of your life.

As long as you allow limiting beliefs to influence your choices, then prosperous living will always seem just out of reach. By applying the techniques you have just been given you can take gigantic steps forward in releasing these patterns and creating powerful new ones that will forge a bright and successful future that will last you a lifetime.

Affirmations for Abundance

- I create abundance easily and effortlessly in everything I have, be, or do.
- With each moment my prosperity increases.
- I make money whether I am awake or asleep.
- I am worthy to receive the abundance of Life.
- Every time I give with joy it comes back to me multiplied
- Every time I receive with joy, I receive more.
- Money comes to me easily and effortlessly.
- All of my moments are filled with richness.
- I am fulfilled and enriched by my work.
- I now live what I love and it works for me.
- I am highly creative, financially thriving, and successful in every way.
- I have all the time in the world to do the things that matter most.
- I am so grateful to have an abundance of health, wealth, and happiness.
- I am abundant.

HERE'S HOW TO SPEND THE NEXT 5 MINUTES

One of the areas that some get stuck in is being open to receive abundance. Life is constantly sending you opportunities to have more of what you want, but are you receptive to them, or are they passing you by because you are distracted by what's going on?

Close your eyes and imagine that you have everything you've ever wanted or needed. See if you can let the 'feeling' of abundance flow through your mind and body. How does it feel to have no wants, needs, or desires anymore? Stay connected to this feeling for a few moments and don't try to change it or control it in any way. Instead, just observe it.

As you allow this space within you to be okay, you are accepting the abundance of life that lives within you and around you. Then, place your hands over your heart and say, "I am so happy that I am abundant in love, health, finances, and joy".

HEALTH AND LONGEVITY

Love That You Live

As I stood talking before a large group of people at one of my seminars, it occurred to me that every change we want to make in our lives has something to do with healing some area of our life.

Whether you want to quit smoking, lose weight, get a new job, or find your perfect partner they all have one thing in common - the desire for something different. If you desire change then what you are really saying is that you are not happy with where you are at. Therefore, the healing that is needed is to turn suffering into joy.

The greatest healing power I have come across is the healing power of love.

More importantly I am speaking of self-love. Self-love is something that appears to elude many. If more people had it there wouldn't be nearly as much pain and suffering in the world.

I've noticed after working with thousands of people that love is something that people find easy to give away but almost impossible to keep.

When I looked deep into my own heart to find the answer for why that was missing in my life, I realized that it never really dawned on me that love was something I had to give to myself.

I'd always thought it was something that I would feel in a relationship or share with those closest to me. But what happens to love when you feel like you simply don't have any more to give or you have trouble receiving it?

Without love in your life - and I'm not talking about the love of others here, I mean the love that fills you up on the inside from your own heart, you will always feel an emptiness that seems impossible to fill.

Many try to fill this emptiness with work, food, addictions, TV, or any multitude of things that distract them from the obviousness that their life is not whole in some way.

Wholeness means learning how to love yourself from the inside-out. This is not something most of us are taught as kids because very few people are living it. Most people choose survival rather than love as their main focus in life, and so the fight to survive and thrive leads them on a long and exhausting path of quiet desperation.

Many go on trying to give meaning to their lives by filling it up with all sorts of things that they think makes them happy or satisfied, only to realize when they go to bed at night that there is a deep emptiness or aloneness inside them that won't go away – no matter what they try and do to hide from it.

We are made up of more space than matter so it makes sense that emptiness is an integral part of who we are.

Loving who you are is a lifelong pursuit. It is something that you need to be mindful to do each day. Like anything, the more love you can find inside you, the more love you will have to enjoy in every part of your life.

HERE'S HOW TO SPEND THE NEXT 5 MINUTES

Loving yourself is perhaps the most important practice of all and, for some their lives will depend upon it. When you're at your breaking point or you feel like you are drowning in misery or emptiness, or even if you just want to have more love in your life than fear. Here's a simple mindfulness technique you can use right now.

As you breathe in, say to yourself, "Breathing in - I love myself", and as you breathe out repeat in your mind, "Breathing out – I am so happy". Then repeat the same phrases with each breath in and out. As you notice other thoughts and feelings arise, just let them come and go without getting attached to them and simply bring your attention back to your breath in and out, and the affirmation you are using.

The reason why you use these words is that by reminding yourself that you are breathing in and breathing out before you repeat your affirmation it helps your mind to be aware of the present moment and not wander away so easily. Because you are already breathing, it just makes this action more conscious and then you add-on the affirmation that is connected with your breath.

Although you can do this for just 5-minutes a day, if you are feeling bad about yourself or life seems to be closing in around you and you are not coping too well, then I would recommend you do this as often as you can. There's no downside to doing it all day long.

In fact, the more you do it, the more you will start to feel good about yourself again. Pretty soon you'll find yourself loving life again and experiencing beautiful things in your life once more.

Your Body is a Temple

The first step to allowing more love in your life is to start treating your body like it's a temple. After all, our bodies are organic in nature and if we constantly fill them with junk food and junk thoughts then are we really giving ourselves the highest love possible?

The physical body is only one part of us that sends us messages of distress and pain. Our mind and feelings also send us warning signals when something is out of balance. There are many ways that these signals can reveal themselves but the most obvious ones are when we notice that something is out of balance mentally, physically, or emotionally.

To ignore these signals is to invite more pain into your life. The best definition I have come across for pain and suffering is:

Suffering = Pain X Resistance to Change

The best part of this formula is that it indicates that any time we experience pain in our life it is a signal that change is required. The more we avoid making changes we instinctively know we need to make, the more suffering we have to endure.

If you think back over your life and recall any time that you were suffering for any reason you will be able to see that it was when you decided to change something you were thinking or doing that eventually brought relief.

A simple example is that if you hate conflict yet find yourself arguing with people all the time and this adds stress to your life; then wouldn't it make sense to just stop being argumentative? This means changing how you communicate including the tone you use, the words you say, and whether you are being aggressive or assertive.

The key factor in the example above is that all that is needed to stop having grief in relationships is to make a change around how you communicate with people. By not making that change, the suffering continues.

Symptom Vs. Cause

It amazes me how modern medicine has come so far in being able to treat such a wide range of pains and illness that plague us yet we are still in the embryo stage of treating what causes these things to happen in the first place.

Take a headache. You can easily pop a headache pill to relieve the discomfort, and as helpful as this may be in the short term, what has the pill done to remove what caused the headache in the first place?

If you can discover what rigid thoughts you are focusing on, what stress and tension you may be hanging on to or what feelings you are suppressing that are causing your headache, then you can stop the behavior that is causing your condition and enjoy a headache-free life.

Doesn't this sound smarter than spending the rest of your life on medication? Don't get me wrong. I am not anti-medicine. I am aware that without it some people's lives would be intolerable. All I am saying is to consider the possibility that you have the power within you to heal much of your life just by changing habits and re-setting your life values.

Pain is our teacher not our torturer. It is a warning signal that something is not right.

Many of us do not heed the warning that pain brings and when that happens, louder and more painful messages are sent. Curing the symptom relieves the immediate pain and suffering. Removing the cause makes sure it doesn't happen again.

The Balancing Act

This is my philosophy on health - practice living a balanced lifestyle. Any area of your life that is not in balance will impact other areas if left unattended. For example, if you are not happy in your work this will eventually have a negative impact in other areas of your life such as your health, relationships, sleep patterns, and self-esteem.

Let us look at some different definitions of health. Some of the dictionary definitions are: *wholeness; fitness; freedom from disease and lack of ailments.* My definition is, *"to live in harmony with your mind, body, and spirit."*

Illness or disease is defined by the dictionary as: *sickness, ill health, ailment, or disorder.*

My definition is, *"focusing on the limiting attributes of the mind or body."*

Many of the illnesses that people experience do not need to happen. The choices that some make about how to live, what to put into their body and how they handle the trials and tribulations of daily living all have an impact on health and longevity.

Your mind only knows what you focus on.
If you focus on imbalance - it will increase.
If you focus on health - it will increase.

That's why learning how to master your mind is a massive step forward in not only helping to heal your body but also in having the best chance at a happy, healthy and long life filled with love and joy.

The Ultimate Diet

Physical health is vitally important to mental and emotional health. Without a healthy body it is almost impossible to deal with negative thoughts and feelings.

Let's look at some more ways of having a body that radiates health and vitality. Many of the foods we eat and things we do with our bodies are purely habitual and have no real value in terms of health and happiness.

Diet consists of three parts:

- **Your mental diet** – this is what you feed your mind.
- **Your physical diet** – what you feed your body.
- **Your emotional diet** – the emotions that rule your life and impact on what you eat, how you think, and how much stress or anxiety you experience.

A healthy mental diet is one that is focused on helping your mind to be calmer, more open, more flexible in attitudes, and that stimulates your imagination and creativity in a positive way. If you do nothing to change the way you think about yourself and life, then you are neglecting the most valuable and powerful resource you have for positive change.

You mind is capable of creating a billion dollar empire, writing books, discovering cures for diseases or any number of new and exciting ventures. On the other hand, if you let it focus on negativity, hardship and drama, you could end up a basket case.

Give your mind more of what it needs to be your best friend who is always there to support you no matter what. All too often when we don't take control of our mind it can make our lives a living hell. One thing you can do to start mastering your mind is to put aside an hour a day to re-educate yourself.

Just like you're reading this book and learning more about who you are and what is possible in your life, reading at least one self-help book a month or listening to a motivational or self-help audio for twenty or thirty minutes each day will make a world of difference.

Throw away the glossy magazines and TV shows filled with trivia and drama, and instead start filling your mind with things that will take you closer to your dream lifestyle.

Your mind is like a garden. You can either plant the seeds of beautiful flowers that will eventually blossom when fed the right nourishment, or you can let weeds take root and kill off all the beautiful flowers before they even grow.

HERE'S HOW TO SPEND THE NEXT 5 MINUTES

Find a self-help book or Podcast that you'd like to read or listen to. Then, spend at least ten to twenty minutes every day reading or listening to it. Just by adding this to your daily rituals you'll soon start to gain new ideas and insights into how you can live a better quality of life.

Healthy Body - Happy Life

It has always made perfect sense to me that if you want optimum health and vitality then start with your physical body. The following guidelines will assist to:

- Detoxify your cells and organs
- Oxygenate the blood
- Improve skin tone
- Improve energy levels and reduce tiredness
- Promote health and longevity
- Super boost your immune system
- Aid digestion

Follow a simple diet that gives you physical energy and supplies your body with what it needs to function efficiently.

Food should be able to be digested quickly. Preparation, serving and cleaning time should be kept to a minimum and be done with joy.

Consume mostly pure and natural foods (that is. organic). Fermented sunflower, almond, or pumpkin seeds are a good source of protein and fiber. There is less energy required to digest this form of protein because it is easily ingested.

193

Soak the seeds in water for eight hours. Drain and blend with filtered water in a food processor until the seeds become paste like. Place into a bowl and cover with a cotton cloth at room temperature for a further eight hours.

Tips to help get the most benefit from your food:

- Eat slowly. Take the time to enjoy the food you are eating. This allows your food to be properly digested.
- Eat for the joy of eating, not as a chore.
- Eat only what you need. Overeating or excessive fasting can place undue stress on your body.
- Toxins create stiffness and stress in the body. Eliminate as many toxic substances as you can from your diet. This includes artificial colors, flavors, and numbers.
- Aim for balance in your diet. Most things in moderation will benefit you greater than too little or too much.

Hydration:

- Drink plenty of filtered water. This assists the body's natural detoxification process.
- Freshly squeezed juice from organic fruit and vegetables is a high source of vitamins and minerals. Consume within seven minutes of juicing, otherwise most of the goodness will have evaporated.

Exercise:

- Pick an exercise that you enjoy and do three lots of twenty minutes a week. Keep a balance between aerobic, muscle tone and stretching whenever possible.
- Strengthening your cardiovascular system allows you to feel more alive and energized.
- Exercise allows your body to efficiently release toxins, your mind to become clearer and more focused and for stress and tension to be dissolved.

Skin Care:

- Use natural products whenever possible to clean your body. Many of the regular cleansing products contain dangerous chemicals such as Sodium Laurel Sulphate (SLS) which are extremely toxic to your body. It's a good idea to understand how to read food and product labels so you identify numbers and ingredients that are potentially harmful.
- Enjoy the experience of touching and being touched. The same as plants respond to loving words and touch so too does your body and skin. Treat them both with tenderness and kindness and you will see and feel the difference.

Super Boost Your Immune System:

- Vitamin and mineral supplements can compensate for what your body may not receive in your diet. Good nutrition is vital, not just for physical health but for mental health as well.

- Get rid of excess stress each day from your body. Exercise is the best way to achieve this. You don't have to exercise for long but make sure it's intense.
- Laugh a little each day. Happiness is the fastest way to heal or stay healthy. The less serious you take yourself and the world around you the lighter your life will be.

HERE'S HOW TO SPEND THE NEXT 5 MINUTES

Take a moment to map out what you are going to do differently from now on to help you achieve peak health and vitality. It may just be one thing that you want to do differently to start with, or it may be more. Make a note of what you are now committing to do to help you to move forward to a happier, healthier, and more productive life.

Putting the Pieces Together

There are many influences that shape our physical, mental, and emotional lives. Diet is just one aspect of a very large jigsaw puzzle. I am constantly amazed at the exceptions to the rules that exist in the world of health.

On one hand you can have someone who drinks alcohol and smokes cigarettes their whole life and lives into their nineties. On the other hand someone who is athletic watches their diet and trains regularly may drop dead from a heart attack at thirty.

This alone proves that there is more to health than just what you eat, drink, or consume. If you take into consideration other factors such as work and living environments, capacity to handle stress and genetic tendencies of your blood line then a bigger picture emerges to be looked at.

Healthy living is really about making a values-based decision to make it a priority in your life regardless of the circumstances. We all have things that we value or prioritize over other things. Some people value work and money more than say diet or exercise, while others value family and friends, more than they value work and money.

Regardless of your intrinsic values, to enjoy more health and vitality it has to be right at the top of your list of things you value.

For me, this means that if I were asked to do something that would add more stress to my life than what I know is healthy for me then I'd decline it – even if there was a huge payday at the end of it. The bottom line is that if something doesn't fit in with my core value of health-first, then it's not going to happen.

Energy Fields

Energy fields are present within animate and inanimate life-forms. A rock for example has an energy field but it is not as easy to detect as that of a plant or animal. Everything that exists is made of energy at some level or another.

The only difference is the level of density or the rate of vibration at which they resonate. A dense object such as rock vibrates at a lower frequency than a lighter object such as water or gas.

Test it out for yourself. The next time you are about to eat something, place your hands a few inches above the food and see if you can feel the energy field emanating from it.

Once you attune your awareness to the differing vibrations of those things you come into contact with each day, you will have a greater appreciation and sensitivity for the life around and within you.

People also have energy fields moving in and around them. This is commonly known as your aura. To become aware of the energy that flows through your body as 'chi' just shake your hands for a few minutes, rub them together with rapid movements and then hold them about 2-3 inches apart and move them slowly towards and away from each other.

If you are doing it correctly you should be feeling magnetic-like energy building up between your hands. See how far you can move your hands apart before you lose awareness of this energy.

If it is not working for you then after shaking your hands, hold your arms out in front of you, stretch your fingers, and then make a tight fist. Do this a few times and then bring your hands together again and repeat the above movement.

Healing Hands

Energy is the source of all life. You can call this energy by any name you like but until you experience for yourself just how far and wide it spreads its wings, then you are missing out on big part of life.

This exercise is an opportunity to get to know a deeper level of love and trust that flows within every cell of your body. When allowed through proper focus and intention, this energy can be harnessed as a tool for manifesting anything you want in life no matter how big or small.

For this exercise you will need a partner. Practice with someone you feel comfortable with at first. For the sake of this exercise you will be called the 'giver' and the person you are working with will be called the 'receiver'. It is best if the receiver either lies down or sits comfortably to assist them to relax deeply during this exercise.

The next step is to close your eyes and take a few moments to relax your body, quiet your mind, and attune your hands to work with energy. Attuning your hands is as easy as imagining that a golden or white light is flowing through the palms of your hands.

If you find it hard to imagine this then simply trust that the moment you ask for healing energy to flow through you, it is instantly made available for you to use. Then, all you need to do is forget about it and let it happen.

After completing the attunement slowly place your hands a few inches from the receiver's body and see if you can feel or sense an energy field coming from their body. It can be experienced in various ways such as:

- Heat
- Magnetic field
- Tingling
- Vibrations
- Cold

Then, allow your hands to gently connect with the receiver's body. It makes no difference whether your hands are slightly above the receiver's body or lightly touching. Let your hands be guided to where the energy is needed most. Your mind may think one thing yet your inner knowing is telling you something different. Trust your instincts.

If your partner has not experienced anything like this before, then spend a few moments explaining the procedure to them. Do everything possible to ensure that they are comfortable, relaxed and at ease before proceeding. This can include making sure the room is warm, lighting is not too bright and having relaxing background music can help.

All you need to do is visualize the energy you are giving as a golden light or feel it as a warm, tingling sensation that flows through your body, into the palms of your hands and extends into the body before you.

Have no expectations about what will happen for the receiver. Just be in the joy of giving unconditionally.

Allow at least five to twenty minutes of focusing on healing energy flowing through you and into the person receiving the healing session. Use this time to relax and let go of any thoughts or concerns you may have gathered during the day.

*The receiver may experience feelings of
heat or energy moving through their body
or they may even feel emotional
and start to laugh or cry.*

These things are all quite natural and there is no need
to be alarmed. Energy is unblocking and emotions are
a natural way to release stuck energy from the body.

If an emotional reaction does eventuate it is even
more important to keep focusing energy through your
palms until the person is at peace again. Most of the
time though the person you are working with will
either fall asleep because they are so relaxed or will
feel a deep calmness yet be highly energized.

When you feel that you are finished, gently lay your
hands on the receiver's shoulders to assist in
grounding them and let them know that when they are
ready, they can open their eyes. Share your
experiences with each other and then swap so that
you are now the receiver and your partner is the giver.

Be sure to advise your partner of the intention of the
exercise and open yourself to receive an abundance
of unconditional love from the universe. When you
have finished receiving, slowly bring your awareness
back to your body and again share your experiences
with each other.

The most common comments expressed by people
who have experienced this technique for themselves
at my seminars and workshops is that they feel:

- Deeply relaxed

- Clarity of mind and thoughts
- Refreshed and energized
- Lighter and 'buzzing' on the inside
- Completely balanced

The upside is that there is no downside to this activity. Absolutely no harm can come from it and what's even better is that the more you practice it, the more energized, peaceful, and alive you will feel.

GOING WITHIN

*The journey of a thousand miles
begins with a single step*

When do you feel the most relaxed? Is it when you watch television, listen to music, soak in a tub, go to bed, or perhaps when the children finally settle down for the night? Are you able to relax deeply or do you find that even though you body may be inactive other parts like your mind are still quite busy?

What most people consider as rest and relaxation is often nothing more than a temporary distraction from the ongoing stress of hectic living. Make no mistake about it - stress kills. If you doubt this then just visit your local hospital and find out what sort of lives seriously ill people have been living.

Stress in relationships, careers, or financial matters, can have devastating results on your physical well-being if it's not dealt with.

One of the most convenient, inexpensive and enjoyable ways to counteract the adverse affects of stress is to meditate.

Meditation is used by millions of people around the world for all sorts of reasons. Some meditate to relax, clear the mind, and ease health issues, while others explore the far reaching benefits that meditation offers in the world of self-development.

One thing's for sure - meditation works. However, it doesn't always work the same way for everyone. What I mean by that is that I have studied more than 120 different meditation techniques over seventeen years and what I've noticed is that there's no such thing as one meditation technique that will work for everyone. In fact, the #1 reason why people give up on meditation all too soon is because they haven't yet found one that works for them.

The point here is that I guarantee there is a meditation technique that will work for you. You just need to keep looking until you find it. Perhaps one of the meditations in this book or from one of my meditation courses which you can do for free will help get you started.

Mediation can be broken down into two main types. These are called active and passive meditation techniques.

An active meditation technique is simply one where you move your body as part of your meditation technique. Even walking, running, dancing, or any type of movement can be used if it is approached in the right way. I have found that most people who lead busy lives and who have never succeeded at meditating before tend to benefit the most from doing active mediations.

A passive meditation technique generally requires starting your meditation from a seated position before settling into a meditative state. The aim of both active and passive meditation techniques is to quiet the mind and allow a deep rest to arise within your mind, body, and emotions.

The mistake many people make when learning to meditate is to have the expectation that they can instantly meditate as deep as a Zen monk. When you think about it a Zen monk has typically been studying meditation for years and their mind and body is conditioned to be quiet and still. While some may find this easy to do, for others it simply won't be possible because their mind won't be quiet and their body becomes agitated.

The best way to approach meditation is to be playful with it and learn to enjoy it as fun.

The great news is that active meditation techniques are not only fun but they work fast. By getting your body involved in the meditation process it helps to slow your mind down and prepare your mind and body for deep relaxation. So if you have had difficulty with sitting still and trying to quiet your mind using passive meditation techniques, then active meditation will be the answer to your prayers.

I Am Stillness Itself

One of the benefits of meditation is to get more in touch with you as the 'human being' rather than just keep plodding along each day stuck in the routine of your 'human doing.'

A 'human doing' is someone who is constantly filling their lives from the outside and forgetting about your being on the inside. In the Western world we are so accustomed to travelling through life at full speed that we often forget to slow down enough to enjoy the ride.

The misconception that many people have is that activity is critical to feel alive or have meaning. I even know people who feel guilty about taking out time to do nothing as they feel like they are wasting time.

There is tremendous power in stilling your mind from the constant energy suck of endless thoughts, feelings and bodily sensations, and being able to find relief from the stress and tensions that they all too frequently bring.

The key to stilling your mind is to live in the moment with deepening awareness of being here now no matter what is going on in or around you.

Interestingly enough, I've also discovered that some people are so preoccupied with their busy lives and the distractions that it provides that a part of them that is not comfortable even at the thought of having a quiet mind and being 'still' for a while.

I know this to be true because I had to confront this within myself. One of the deepest fears that I uncovered many years ago was the fear of being alone. For me, I had no idea what my 'being' even felt like, let alone knew where or how to look for it. I was so programmed to go, go, go in my life that I never realized I was on the fast-track to burning out.

At this time in my life I had a high-flying corporate job at an international airline and was travelling all the time. However, even though I was always busy, meeting new people and visiting new and exciting places, there was still a nagging feeling of emptiness or something missing in my life.

The turning point happened for me when one day I was walking along a track in a magnificent forest and I was drawn to lie down and rest underneath a giant oak tree.

I lay there staring up into the sky watching the leaves dancing in the wind. Time seemed to slow down and stand still. My mind went very quiet, so quiet in fact that it felt like it was completely empty of thoughts. This was my first experience e of what I call 'stillness'.

It's a little hard to describe what stillness feels like inside you but image what it would be like to feel totally at peace with life. It's like time stood still and there was nothing else needed apart from the blissful experience of being here and now.

When your mind is still a calmness and peacefulness arises inside you. Then you can see things clearly and life gets easier.

I now know that every single one of us can access this same place inside us. All that is needed is to quiet your mind for a moment and then you will be able to experience the bliss of stillness for yourself.

HERE'S HOW TO SPEND THE NEXT 5 MINUTES

Here's a way that you may be able to trick your mind into becoming still for a moment.

Place a candle in front of you so that the flame is level with your eyes. Your body is comfortable and your spine is straight. With your eyes open, gaze at the flame. Do not blink - just look. Blinking means thinking. Your look is soft and aware, not tense or forced. Keep your eyes as still as possible and let your gaze gently penetrate into the flame.

At first your eyes may water and feel a little uncomfortable. This is a natural reaction and there is nothing to be afraid of. This is a part of a cleansing process that will benefit you greatly. Eventually, you will forget that you are looking at the candle and in that moment a gap is created in your thoughts and you will experience the stillness of 'no mind'.

Do this meditation for at least five minutes a day, preferably before you go to sleep or in the morning when you awake. If you apply this technique as soon as you get up you will notice a tremendous improvement in the quality of your day. If applied just before sleep, you will wake up feeling more refreshed and relaxed and your dreams will have a new dimension added to them.

An alternative to this is to simply focus on a dot or spot on a wall until it disappears. This is a great meditation to do if you are having difficulty letting go of the day or you are suffering from insomnia. It will also help you to focus your mind like a laser beam, which will bring many benefits to your home and work life.

Meditation Techniques for Busy People

On one level meditation has helped me to let go of fear and anxiety while opening to deeper levels of calmness and joy. On another level it has helped to find my life's purpose, get in touch with my spirit, and live a life that I absolutely love to wake up to each and every day.

If you are a bit skeptical that something so apparently simple as meditation could do these things, then don't be concerned because I was the biggest skeptic of all when I got started. There's nothing wrong with having doubts about anything as it just means that you have a questioning mind – and that's always a good thing.

When it comes to meditation I always recommend that you trust your own instincts. Be skeptical if you need to be, but don't let that stop you from exploring the possibility that there may be something in it for you.

There are so many benefits mentally, physically, emotionally, and spiritually to meditation that it would take an entire book to cover them all.

So what exactly is meditation? I call it the art of doing nothing. By this I mean for some of us sitting silently and doing nothing is incredibly hard to do. I know this was true for me in the beginning because I had places to be and things to do, so being able to relax and enjoy being here now was not so easy.

That's why I call it an art. Because like anything, if we really want to master it, then we need to practice it until it becomes second nature. The more silent you can be in your mind and body, the deeper your meditations will be.

Meditation is what happens when you have finished a meditation technique and you find yourself being completely silent and still in both your mind and body.

In other words, we first need to 'do' something with our mind or body by using an active or passive meditation technique to prepare us for meditation to happen.

That's why meditation techniques were created; to help you to quiet your mind, so that your body can relax and you can be comfortable just 'being' for a few moments. After all, we are human beings and we tend to forget to honor the 'being' part of us as we get lost in the never ending treadmill of doing.

Meditation is free, requires no special equipment or skills, and can be done almost anywhere and at any time.

Here are some simple meditation techniques that you can try any time you want as they all have a slightly different focus and will bring a variety of mental, physical, and emotional benefits into your life. Never treat meditation seriously as it is meant to be playful. The more fun you have learning it and doing it, then you will be surprised how your meditation will grow in leaps and bounds.

Breathing Meditation

This is one of the simplest and most effective techniques to get started with. It just takes a few minutes and can be done almost anywhere and at any time. It's great for clearing your mind, bringing you fully into the present moment, and giving your energy levels an instant spike.

The technique is simple. Just be conscious of breathing in and breathing out. If you are visual then as you breathe in imagine that you are watching your breath come into your body and all the way town to your belly.

Then as your breathe out, watch it move back up through your body and out through your mouth. If you are not visual, then try and imagine or feel the movement of your breath in and out.

When we are tense or anxious our breathing becomes shallow, which disconnects us from our body and causes tension and stress to build up in our muscles and joints.

The simple act of conscious breathing allows you to connect to your body, get you out of your head, and bring you into the present. It is without a doubt the quickest way to dissolve tension and relax your mind and body.

Practice this technique daily, anytime that you become aware that you are feeling tired, drained, tense, or flustered. It will instantly connect you to your body and help get rid of stress and tension.

This is also a great way to start the day so that you are centered and relaxed and especially to end the day so you can clear out your mind and body from the events of the day.

Clearing Your Mind

This is a simple technique for rapidly clearing your mind and emotions and putting your body into an energized state. It is also a great way to release toxins from your body through your breath. You can do it for any length of time from a few minutes to as long as you like.

Stage One: *Counting Your Breath*

The basis of this technique is for each breath you take in you will be breathing out for double the amount of time. So if your breath in is for five seconds, then you will breath out is for ten seconds.

To start with, let you breath flow naturally into your body through your nose. Only breathe in as much as you would in a normal resting position. As you breathe in start counting in your head from the number one to whatever number you get to by the time your lungs are full.

Then, remember what number you got to (that is, 10) and then very slowly release your breath through your mouth. The aim is to breathe out until you get to double the number you counted for your breath in (that is, 20).

Continue to breathe like this for five minutes, preferably in a sitting position. The purpose in breathing this way is to help release toxins and 'old' energy from your body. It is a great way to feel more relaxed, energized, and alive.

Stage Two: *Lie Down and be Still*

At the end of the time let your breathing return to normal and allow yourself to sit quietly for another few minutes. Keep your eyes closed during this stage. You can also lie down and relax if that is more comfortable.

Improving Your Focus

This is a fixed gazing meditation technique that can be used to develop concentration, strengthen your eyes, improve memory, and clear your mind. By fixing your gaze, the restless mind will eventually stop. I am able to hold my gaze for 45 minutes at a time without blinking now but this took a while to achieve. Start off with what is comfortable for you and then increase it slowly over time if you want to experience even more benefits.

Stage One: *Fixed Eye Gazing*

In a seated position fix your attention on a single point such as a candle flame or a black dot in the middle of a white sheet of paper. Make sure that it's at eye level and about three to four feet away. Simply gaze at the candle flame or black dot and if any thought's or feelings arise, acknowledge them and then gently bring your awareness back to the object of your focus. Continue to gaze at the object until your eyes begin to water. Then close them and relax. The longer you can gaze without blinking, the clearer and more focused your mind will become.

Stage Two: *Be Still*

Close your eyes. Sit or lie down and be still for 15 minutes.

Boost Your Productivity

Meditation techniques to help improve focus and productivity get the best results when you practice them on a regular basis. It's a lot like a fitness program for your mind, where each rep you do strengthens your attention and improves your ability to focus. When life is hectic and there's no time to think clearly and your to-do list just keeps piling up, then it's almost impossible to do things properly or well. This is when productivity drops off.

This is a simple form of mindfulness meditation. Just sit in a comfortable position on a chair or on the floor for five minutes. Make sure your back is relatively straight. Close your eyes and relax your body. Let your awareness move inside and observe your breathing. There's no need to change your breathing; just watch it. Feel the actual sensations of your breathing and when your mind goes away to something else just bring your mind back to being aware of your breathing.

Get in Touch With Your Heart

Settle into a comfortable position and ensure that your spine is as straight as possible. Close your eyes and visualize that you have no head. There is only an empty space where your head used to be. Now imagine, and if you can feel, that you are breathing in through the center of your chest.

Without a head, your thoughts will naturally drop to your heart area. With each heartbeat, feel your thoughts dissolving into the warmth and love emanating from the relaxing inner rhythm of your beating heart.

Imagine or feel the blissful union of your thoughts merging with your heartbeat. Experience the

216

freedom of the empty space above your shoulders and let life flow to and from your heart, without a mind to create tension.

Feel your body relaxing even deeper as you radiate love both within and around you. Allow this love to expand into every cell of your body.

Then, when you have finished and you are at peace once again you can put your head back on your shoulders if you like. There is no minimum or maximum time limit for this meditation.

Whenever you find yourself stressed by negative thoughts, stop whatever you are doing and do this simple meditation technique. It will have an immediate calming influence upon you and life will once again become heartfelt and simple.

The beauty of this meditation is that you can do it almost anywhere and anytime. You can practice this meditation while talking to others, walking down the street, or any time you wish to relax and live life from your heart, not your head.

Just For Couples

This is a very beautiful meditation that will create a deeper intimacy with your partner and allow for a beautiful connection based on openness, trust, and allowance.

Firstly, sit opposite your partner making sure that you are both comfortable and at the same height. Keep the lighting low and make sure you will not be disturbed. Secondly, gaze into each other's eyes.

Do not be alarmed if your partner's face starts to change or you lose sight of the eyes completely. This is quite natural and means that you are gazing beyond normal vision.

As soon as you start gazing into each other's eyes focus on breathing in unison. Synchronize your breath in and out as if you are one person. At the same time stay focused on each other's eyes. Let your gaze be soft and relaxed and you are breathing as natural as possible.

At the end of this meditation come together and connect with each other in whatever way you like physically. Do your best to maintain the beautiful space you created between you during the meditation while you come together physically.

Walking With Mindfulness

Stage One: *Walking*:

Go for a walk somewhere that you enjoy. If possible walk along the beach or where there are trees and flowers. Walk slowly and let your body relax. Your breath is kept relaxed and easy. Let your eyes enjoy the colors of the flowers, the beauty of the trees, the ocean, or even the sky.

Let your ears enjoy the sounds of nature or of soothing music if you are wearing headphones. Bring your awareness to your feet and connect with how your feet feel as they connect with the ground. Be aware of the difference of the various surfaces on your feet and how they feel and sound as you walk.

Stage Two: *Be Still*

Sit for a while with your back against a tree, or on something comfortable on the ground. You can even lie down if you like. Allow any tension to sink out of your body and into the ground. Close your eyes and be still for a few minutes.

Sleep Well

If you find it hard to sleep it is usually because of an overactive mind. This comes from an accumulation of energy that gets stored in the body during the day. Before you can fall asleep easily you must first find a way to release pent up energy that is often held onto as tension in your body. It is these tensions that keep you awake.

Here is a meditation technique that will help you to fall asleep easily:

1. Make a regular time to go to bed and stick to it as best you can. This helps your body get into a rhythm.
2. Before going to bed do fifteen minutes of vigorous dancing to help release any tension in your body. The more you throw yourself into the dancing, the more tension you will get rid of and the easier you will fall asleep.
3. As soon as you have stopped dancing then have a hot bath and let your body relax for ten to fifteen minutes and let the hot water soothe the tensions out of your body as you relax in the bath. If you don't have a bath, then have a hot shower.
4. Finally, have a hot drink. Nothing with caffeine in it of course. Hot milk or some herbal tea will do nicely.
5. Then go to bed and sleep. Make sure that the previous steps were all completed before your regular bed time as these must be done as part of your preparation for sleep.

Meditation and Manifesting Your Destiny

Meditation is just like any other practice such as yoga, Tai Chi, going to the gym, cardio, learning a new skill, cooking, or anything at all that you want to become good at - it requires practice.

Yes, it can be used for a 'quick fix' from stress-related symptoms but that is just the surface of what meditation can do. From helping you to stay calm and centered, and be clear-headed most of the time, through to opening your brain to higher levels of creativity and being more productive and effective in your life, meditation is a gift that keeps on giving the more you use it.

I have found that by putting aside five minutes at the end of each meditation to focus on what I want to attract into my life, that this accelerates results. It's the perfect time to do your affirmations and visualizations of exactly how you want your personal or professional life to be.

The reason why this is the best time to visualize how you want your life to be is because you are already in a relaxed state, your mind is clearer, and your brain is functioning at the optimum level for attracting to you what you want.

If you want a pay raise, then focus on seeing yourself getting it at the end of your meditation. If you want to find your soul mate then picture yourself with the person of your dreams. If you simply want to be at peace with your life, then let this be the focus of your integration period.

Always visualize your desired destiny as if it's actually already happening to you right now. Make it real in your mind; make it detailed. Enter the role and become it in your mind.

Never have any expectation of 'when' your object of desire will come to fruition – that is not the point of the exercise. The purpose is to tell your brain how you want your life to be as if it already exists and to keep imprinting this image over and over again for weeks or months until it turns up in your life.

The bottom line is that any thought you put into your mind at the end of your meditation, and it is regularly nourished, will produce results in your life.

If you want to see how this works in practice then grab this free guided meditation series on the link below:

www.MasterYourMindspace.com/meditationprogram

EASY DOES IT

We look at it and do not see it;
its name is the invisible.

We listen to it and do not hear it;
its name is the inaudible.

We touch it and do not find it;
its name is the subtle.

"The Way of Lao-tzu"

Is there is anything you could be doing differently in your life to allow your journey to be filled with more ease and less struggle?

One weekend I went four-wheel driving in a remote part of Northern Australia. After several hours of driving along narrow dirt roads, I began to be concerned about the degenerating conditions of the track I was following.

Recent rain had caused extensive flooding and the further along the track I went, the muddier it became.

I had been heading inland towards a remote river to spend the day swimming, camping, and relaxing. Off

to my right I could just make out a small section of the river winding its way through dense bush.

At the same time the wheels of my four wheel drive started slipping and sliding in the thickening mud. I was only about one kilometer away from my destination, but the road was rapidly losing its appeal to me.

As I slowed to a snail's pace I saw for the first time that I was completely surrounded by swamp. This was enough to make my mind up for me. I had to go back or risk being stuck out here in the middle of nowhere, indefinitely.

There was absolutely nowhere to turn my vehicle around. In every direction there was nothing but more water and mud. I slowed to a complete halt to consider my options and as soon as my four wheel drive stopped moving it sank up to the doors in thick, black mud.

A momentary panic filled me. I was hours by car from the nearest main road, an afternoon tropical storm was approaching, and the only solid ground was several hundred meters behind me.

I looked around and decided to fill the mud track behind me with loose timber and rocks. This was not going to be easy in the heat, mud, and water. I could have left the car where it was and walked back to dry ground, but I was determined not to leave it.

This turned out to be back-breaking work in the sweltering heat and humidity. Inevitably, this idea failed. After spending several hours digging, carrying and filling, all that happened was my vehicle slid sideways into even deeper mud.

Exhausted, out of ideas and dehydrated I dragged myself to the nearest shady tree and collapsed beneath it. I no longer cared enough to struggle with the car anymore. So I decided to forget about it and set off by foot in the direction I had just come from.

I knew it could take a day or two to get to the main road but I had no other choice. It was highly unlikely that another vehicle would come this way for perhaps days.

I reasoned that at the worst, I would have to walk for a few days to get help and at the best there may be other four wheel drivers in this neck of the woods. This last thought cheered me up, so I set off on foot towards dry land with this vision firmly fixed in my mind.

Less than half an hour later I spotted dust on the horizon and soon heard the friendly sound of engines heading my way. Within another couple of hours my vehicle had been safely towed out of the mud and I was joyously heading on my way back home.

This lesson taught me that even when the going gets tough it is far better to relax and enjoy the ride, than it is to get bogged down by panic and fear. The solutions to our challenges are not always obvious but one thing is for sure, if you get stuck focusing on the problem, the solution may just ease on by unnoticed.

Everything Is Great!

The ability to see life through the eyes of innocence and simplicity is one of the most precious gifts anyone can be blessed with. We are all born with this gift, yet time and circumstances inevitably weave a complex web of mistrust and cynicism that causes us to forget the wonderment and countless blessings that surround us.

It happened that a great Maharaja in India ruled with unbending pomposity. The Maharaja's personal advisor was a very wise man and often the Maharaja would seek counsel from him.

One day, the Maharaja received news that a warring tribe of bandits was approaching the palace and he quickly sent for his advisor. When the advisor arrived the Maharaja informed him of the situation and asked him for his counsel.

The advisor laughed and said, *"My lord, this is great news!"*

The Maharaja looked at him absurdly and shouted, *"Have you gone mad? What is great about our palace being in grave danger?"*

"We are blessed to have received advance warning", smiled the advisor calmly. *"You can use this opportunity to bring your people together to fight for a common cause. There will be much rejoicing when the threat to our peaceful nation has been destroyed and your popularity will grow many-fold."*

So it came to pass. The bandits were ambushed by the Maharaja's guards and the celebration lasted for days.

The Maharaja also loved to go hunting and did so once a week no matter what state of affairs called to him. On the next royal hunting day the Maharaja slipped off his mount as he was preparing to ride out, landed heavily on his right arm, and broke it.

The Maharaja cried out in agony as pain exploded up his arm. The advisor, who was nearby, ran over to the Maharaja and proclaimed, *"Your majesty this is great. God is always blessing us with his grace!"*

The Maharaja was so enraged by this that he ordered the advisor to be immediately thrown into the deepest, darkest, and dirtiest dungeon for one week without food or water. The hunting party still went out that day without the Maharaja.

While they were hunting for tigers the Maharaja's soldiers were ambushed by surviving bandits and they were all slaughtered. When the Maharaja heard of this he immediately had his advisor released from prison and brought before him.

The Maharaja looked thoughtfully at his advisor before saying, *"I understand now why you said that breaking my arm was great and that I was blessed by God. If I had been with the hunting party I would have also been killed. This tragedy I could not have foreseen. Something puzzles me though. If you can find something great about every experience what possible blessing did you receive from being thrown in the dungeon?"*

"Oh my Lord!" exclaimed the wide-eyed advisor. *"I am deeply blessed by this experience. If I had not been under arrest I too would have been ordered to go with the hunting party and been killed!"*

Do not be too hasty to condemn your experiences. There is always a light at the end of the tunnel, no matter how dark it may appear to be while you are traveling through it.

Even the darkest hours can bring us new strength and confidence that can lighten our stride and carry us beyond any hardship.

Simple Mind – Simple Life

In the acclaimed film, Forrest Gump, Tom Hanks portrays the essence of purity in the way he approaches life. In his own offbeat way, Gump consistently made the best of where he was and what life brought to him. Sometimes he looked awkward and clumsy, but in many ways he was a master in disguise.

This movie contains a powerful message of unconditional love. Gump rarely had a reason for doing the things he did. His ability to focus and stay focused on what he was doing revealed an uncluttered mind and an ability to live joyfully without expectations.

Gump accepted everything that happened, questioned nothing, and never allowed himself to be dragged down by what life sent to him. He also demonstrated the spiritual qualities of forgiveness, integrity, humility, and compassion.

Gump never had the mindset to tell himself that the things he did were not possible. The benefit was that he was not created any self-imposed limitations to what he could have, be, or do. Instead of looking at life through the eyes of fear, he looked through eyes of love and acceptance.

Whether you look at life through the eyes of fear or love will depend upon who is looking. When your mind is at peace and your heart is open then you can see clearly. Otherwise, the world is colored by whatever glasses (beliefs) you are wearing.

Purity of heart and mind happens when you give up the struggle to find happiness and accept that where you are now is perfect. No matter what life has sent to challenge you, the simpler you live your life, the happier you will be.

If you deal with all things that come upon you with a sense of humor and the willingness to transform your life for the better, then you will never lack for anything.

After all, *"Life is like a box of chocolates - you never know quite what you are going to get."*

HERE'S HOW TO SPEND THE NEXT 5 MINUTES

Pick one of the meditations in the previous pages and then find a quiet and comfortable place to sit where you won't be disturbed for a few minutes.

After you have finished your meditation technique, take a few moments to lie down and just be. During this time you are simply relaxing and letting go of the need to be anywhere or do anything other than be here now.

YOU HAD IT ALL THE TIME

When self improvement gives way to wisdom

I love to learn more about life, love, happiness, and living my full potential while here on earth. In fact, I have been a student of self improvement for more than half my life and have probably invested more than half a million dollars in self education – and if I had my time again I'd do exactly the same.

Here's the thing though… at some point it's time to stop looking for answers and instead start applying what you're learning. That's when knowledge becomes wisdom. For me, that's when everything changed and I began to live a richer, fuller, and more enjoyable life.

Then, at some point a new understanding began to awaken within me. The understanding was that everything I had been learning and doing was all leading me to the same place – me.

Let me explain it this way. When you think about the things that drive you to do the things you do to make a living and enjoy your life what is the real motivation behind your actions?

Is it so that you have more money in the bank, or have more love in your relationships, or have more security and peace of mind in your life? The answer to all of these is of course – yes.

However, what I've discovered is that all of us are driven by one very powerful desire and that desire is to be happy. Regardless of the goals we have, the purpose of any goal is who we become along the way to achieving it and how we feel when we get there.

Whether your goal is to make a million dollars, lose weight, travel more, have more freedom in life, or even just to stop stressing about things, the outcome that all these things will give to you once you have achieved them – is happiness.

Through the miracle of meditation I have come to know that happiness, or joy as it is also known, is something that we have unlimited amounts inside us. The irony is that we don't need to go chasing one dream after another in order to have it – we have it all the time.

What's really obvious to me now is that in the past I used to be focused exclusively on my life in the world, which of course pulls you in a thousand directions each day depending on what's going on. One moment you are sailing smoothly and everything feels great and then the next something happens that throws your equilibrium right out the window.

For me, it meant that happiness was something I experienced when something 'good' happened or I was excited about something I was really looking forward to. The rest of the time, happiness seemed like a long lost relative that may never show up again.

Meditation has shown me that happiness is always there and all that is needed is for my mind to quiet down and my body to be relaxed. You see, I discovered that by being pre-occupied all the time with my busty life, I wasn't taking the time to let my inner peace and happiness come to the surface. It kept getting pushed away because there was no 'space' for it to exist as I went from one distraction to the next.

I share this with you to give you another way to think about happiness and just how beautiful your life could be if that was your priority instead of whatever is pulling you away from it moment to moment. All you need to do is stop moving your mind and body for even 30 seconds and you'll start to feel the peacefulness wash over you and then the joy start to move into every cell of your body.

We have an unlimited supply of happiness and peace at our disposal waiting to be enjoyed – all it takes is to stop running around like a lunatic for a moment and just be. Where are we rushing to anyway that's so important that we'd rather sacrifice our true nature for the promise of an illusory future that may or may not ever happen?

One thing's for sure, if you take the time to just be for twenty minutes a day, you'll soon come to know that you are the happiness and peace that you have always yearned for and the best part is that you don't have to go anywhere or do anything special to enjoy it – because you had it all the time!

Courage – The Joy of Living Dangerously

When I was ten years old I ran away from home. In my mind I was convinced that my parents didn't care about me so my friend John and I decided to run away together. Our plan was pretty simple. We would meet outside John's house at 2.00am and head off into the wilderness.

As the time approached for me to rendezvous with John, I packed a few belongings into my school bag and tiptoed quietly down the hall to the front room. I gingerly opened the front door and sucked my breath in as the chilled night air brought tears to my eyes as it hit my face and cheeks.

Even at the door, a part of me wished that my parents would catch me and scold me for my rash behavior. To my young mind that would have at least proved to me that they cared. As I silently closed the front door behind me I felt a mixture of excitement and sadness.

By the time I had traveled the few blocks to John's house, the cold wind and inky darkness of the night had already started to weaken my resolve.

I had never done anything like this before and a part of me was gloating over the fact that it would serve my parents right when they found me missing. While this thought reassured me, close behind was the thought of how much trouble I would get into if I was ever caught.

To my surprise John was not waiting for me at our prearranged spot. I cautiously made my way around to the back of his house and tapped lightly on his bedroom window. There was no response.

The noise of my fingers tapping on the window pane sounded like cannons going off in the still night air. I was sure that John's parents were going to hear me and then I would have an awful lot of explaining to do.

After several more long and fearful minutes and not so delicate taps on the window, John's face appeared from behind the glass.

With eyes that were filled with sleep he grumbled, *"What do you want?"*

"Don't you remember we are running away tonight?" I hurriedly reminded him.

"I'm too tired," John replied groggily. *"You'd better go home before dad wakes up."*

I stood there for a moment feeling ridiculous. A part of me was relieved because I too was tired and hungry, while another part of me felt let down and disappointed. Feeling confused and frightened, I huddled in an old abandoned shed for a while hoping that my parents might realize I was gone. At least I could return with them knowing how unhappy I was.

This was one of the longest nights of my life. The walls of the shed creaked loudly in the blanket of darkness and the cool winter air whistled eerily through every hole and gap it could find. As the sun started to rise over the horizon, I gratefully unraveled my freezing body from its fetal position and eagerly made my way back home.

When I arrived home the house was in silence. No one was even up yet. I went into my room and fell into a long, deep sleep. Later that day, when I awoke and went into the living room where my parents were, everything was as it always had been.

No one ever knew of my adventure or feelings at that time. I kept this secret to myself as I learned to do with most things in my life.

Many years later I realized that it wasn't that my parents didn't love me. It was that their way of showing love was different from the way I needed to receive it as a child. Because I had no idea how to handle such powerful emotions like feeling unloved, it just seemed easier to try and run away from them.

The same can be said for running away from anything in life that you'd rather not face. It doesn't matter where you go, you will carry your unresolved issue with you, and it will still need to be faced sooner or later.

YOU HAD IT ALL THE TIME

I now know that by moving towards challenges and having the courage to face my fears and insecurities, instead of trying to avoid them, that I resolve things faster and reclaim my personal power with each step forward.

HERE'S HOW TO SPEND THE NEXT 5 MINUTES

Is there something in your life you have been avoiding of late? If so, now is the time to muster up your courage and move towards it.

Take the next few minutes to think about how you are going to approach your situation and then set a date that you are going to take the bull by the horns and tackle it.

Then, take a moment to close your eyes and picture yourself successfully resolving your challenge. If there are people involved, then picture them smiling and nodding their heads in a gesture of acceptance as they say thanks and shake your hand in appreciation.

Caverns of the Soul

While travelling through the United States on a six-month trip I met up with some amazing people and discovered some outrageous places that had a big impact on me.

One particular experience that struck a deep chord happened during a guided tour through a cave in a particular mountain that was open to tourists. The only way to get to the cave was via a cable car that ran almost vertically up the side of the mountain.

236

The tour guide boasted that this was the steepest cable ride in the world and as my body lay pinned uncomfortably against the back of the narrow wooden bench seat, I had no reason to doubt it.

A group of us, led by an energetic young guide, entered into the enormous mouth of the cave and proceeded to follow a string of pale lights above our head that trailed in a downward direction into a silent world of darkness.

After about an hour of exploring the cave our guide stopped for a moment and asked us to stand still and be perfectly quiet. Then, without warning, the lights above our heads went out. My first impression was of isolation. The darkness was unlike anything I had experienced before. It was like a thick inky blackness that was overwhelming.

I could feel my eyes straining to make out an image or object but to no avail. With the lights still off, the guide informed us that within a few days of being lost in such darkness people can go blind and after a week they can go completely insane.

While it's scary to be lost in the darkness that envelopes our lives from time to time, unlike the cave there is always a light to be found. It may not always be obvious yet still it exists. With every fear we overturn and every dark place in our life that we bring a light to, we walk in a brighter world.

The voice of our fears can sometimes be so loud telling us that everything is doom and gloom, but when you turn around and face them head on, then they no longer lurk in the darkness as some faceless unseen demon. Instead, the light of your attention on them sees them instantly starting to fade and the more you look at them and keep moving forward the more their power diminishes.

Our fears would have us believe that we are small and weak. Nothing could be further from the truth. There is nothing small or weak about us except what we imagine to be true. You are perfect as you are and are 100% unique to life. There is no one like you and there never will be again.

Our mission in life is to give ourselves permission to shine the light of our brilliance, joy, and love brighter than any star in the sky. This is how we become liberated from our fears and this is how we help others to do the same.

HERE'S HOW TO SPEND THE NEXT 5 MINUTES

Where do you believe that you are small or weak or don't deserve to have, be, or do something that's important to you? Is there something you've always wanted to do, or someone you need to say something to that you've been holding back on?

If so, take action on it right now. Whether that's to find out what you need to do to get started on something you've been putting off, or if you need to pick up the phone and call someone to share something that's been eating away at you – take a few minutes to do something about it right now. To shine more of your light in the world you have to be willing to shine it wherever you find that doubt and fear exists. Only then will your light get brighter.

The Path of Love

We have talked about loving yourself more as a way to bring more happiness, peace, prosperity, and purpose into your life. Many people seem to struggle with this concept especially if they are going through tough times.

The good news is that there are some practical ways that you can let more love into your life. The first of those ways is to let more love in. This means that whenever you are offered something, be it support, a compliment or even a hug, find a way to say "yes" and be grateful for what you are being given.

I meet people who complain that they don't have enough time, money, or emotional support, and then when these gifts are offered to them, they refuse them.

My aunt regularly complained about how she never got any help around the house. When I offered to organize a house cleaner for her once a week she turned me down flat.

There are two parts to love. It can be given and it can be received. Consider the possibility that if you are not open to do both equally, then it will be hard for the unlimited gifts that love brings for you to rejoice in them.

Over the next 24 hours allow anything that is freely offered to you to be received with gratitude. Life wants to send you more love and the way to open the door is to say "yes" to as many things being given as you can. In every moment there is an opportunity for us to receive more love. It can be found in the wind, the sun, a glass of water or even a kind gesture. Be sure not to let love pass you by again by keeping your mind, heart, and arms open wide.

Radical Forgiveness

The second step on the path of love is to do with self forgiveness. Most of us think about forgiveness in terms of applying it to people who have hurt us in some way or another. Yet as long as we hold on to any past transgressions we are really just hurting ourselves.

To hold on to anything painful from the past or present requires a lot of energy. This can be anything from relationship problems through to any number of mental, physical, or emotional wounds created by mental, physical, emotional pain or abuse.

There is great peace in forgiveness, especially when we apply it to ourselves.

This was an area I struggled with for a long time because of pride and deep seated belief that I was not okay. I was very hard on myself when I made mistakes and was my own worst critic when it came to letting others down or making stupid decisions. On the other hand, it had always been easy for me to

240

forgive and forget the mistakes of others, but I just didn't know how to apply it to myself.

The turning point came when I did a workshop on radical forgiveness. In this workshop we formed a large circle and one by one we had to walk across the circle and say in a loud clear voice whatever was unspoken inside us to forgive.

Obviously, this was quite confronting but such a sacred space was formed between us all by the facilitator, that it made it easy to open up to old wounds and let them out. This process went on for most of the day. We continued to walk across the circle, sharing whatever came up for us over and over again, until we could walk across with our heads held high and power in our voice and body.

This process blew me away. It made me realize just how hard I had been on myself and how much healing I needed to feel really good about myself. What it also proved to me was that no matter how deeply wounded we are from the past, or how deep our problems might be with ourselves, or others, they can be dissolved in an instant if we are ready to let them go.

It didn't take me years to work through my past issues; it happened immediately. Since then, I have discovered that this exact process works for me just by using it with myself in the mirror, or sitting quietly before I go to bed each night and forgiving myself for anything that I might have been hanging on to from the day that was still disturbing me.

Sometimes, forgiving yourself means taking action and sometimes it doesn't. You will know the difference as it is really a judgment call on whether you need to share something with another or not.

The thing to keep in mind if you do involve others is that it is not their place to heal you. That is up to you. They may or may not receive it in the way you imagined so the rule of thumb is that if you do have something to share, make sure that it's absolutely necessary and you have no expectation of how they will react.

HERE'S HOW TO SPEND THE NEXT 5 MINUTES

It's time to do some healing work on yourself. Take a moment to close your eyes and think about something in your past or present that you are holding on to that is causing pain or struggle in your life mentally, emotionally, or physically.

Now put your hands over your heart and say to yourself, "I forgive myself for holding on to (whatever the experience was) and continuing to cause myself pain." You can say this once or as many times as you like until you can say without any negative emotional attachment.

Once you have forgiven yourself, then it becomes infinitely easier to forgive others. It's like anything we do. It's always easier to extend our hand towards others in compassion when we have already extended that same hand in kindness to ourselves.

Think back on those times that someone has told you that it was okay when you made a mistake and didn't try to belittle or make you feel guilty. How did that feel?

This is the exact feeling that you will be bestowing upon others when you let them know that they are okay even though they may have messed up. As the saying goes, *"To err is human; to forgive is Divine"*. The moment you extend your forgiveness outwardly, you will also simultaneously receive more peace and happiness in your life.

Recently, I received a call from my financial advisor who was helping me to get a multi-million dollar business loan for a project I was working on.

I could hear the nervousness in Jane's voice as she anxiously explained to me that the sizeable deposit I had used to initiate the loan process had been embezzled by an accountant she personally knew who was putting the loan together. It wasn't just my money either as he had run off with a bunch of other people's money as well.

Listening to Jane's trembling apology, I could sense that she was waiting for me to unload on her.

"Okay, tell me more about what happened." I asked in a calm voice.

Then she went on to explain what she knew about the embezzlement and that the police were involved. An investigation had already begun and she felt guilty because she had advised me to invest with this particular company.

"You know Jane," I replied, *"I don't blame you for this at all. It's O.K."*

You could have heard a pin drop as I heard Jane breathe a sigh of deep relief. As we hung up, I felt upset that I had money embezzled, yet I felt the most rewarding feeling knowing that I didn't project my disappointment on Jane and that I'd chosen to show her appreciation rather than anger. The result was that there was a peace and calmness between us that could have been potentially destroyed.

244

When we make peace more important than being right or needing to shame, or put others down, we are living forgiveness in action. Yes, we can feel hurt and have things going on for us internally that need to be dealt with, but when we choose to not project them onto others no matter how much we want to, then we are not unnecessarily adding to more pain and suffering in the world – in fact we help it to heal.

HERE'S HOW TO SPEND THE NEXT 5 MINUTES

If there is anyone you have not yet forgiven for a past or present experience, then now is the time to do so. If they are easy to reach, then make a time to go and meet with them and tell them that you forgive them.

If this person is not easy to contact, or perhaps they have passed on from this world, then it can still be done. Sit in a chair and put another chair in front of you. Then close your eyes and invite them to energetically come and sit in the vacant chair. Now speak to them as if they are physically present and tell them that you forgive them.

This is a very powerful exercise and whether they are present or not it's a very effective way to heal relationships.

THE BEST IS YET TO COME

Every Ending Heralds a New Beginning

I think it's safe to say that by now you get the idea that the big secret to mastering your mind-space is to simply find a way that works for you to quiet your mind and be-here-now. It's so easy to get lost in our thoughts and lives that we forget that it's the simplest of things that can help us to find peace, clarity, and happiness.

If you get nothing else from this book but the desire to learn how to still your mind and relax your body deeply every single day for just a few minutes, then you have gained everything I was hoping for when I set out to write it.

There are so many ways to take these ideas, stories, and techniques and apply them to life situations beyond what they were intended for here. Even if you picked just one of the meditation techniques and used it every day for a month, the possibilities of what this could do to bring more happiness, peace, well-being, and vitality is endless.

You've also discovered that focusing on doing something to help change your life for just five minutes a day can make a tremendous difference to the quality of your life. In fact, it's a great daily habit to get into. Then, as you continue to use a technique or meditation that is getting results for you, you can easily increase the amount of time you devote to it.

Now that you've come to the end of this book, it's time to apply what you have learned and start a new chapter in your life. One filled with happiness and peace, passion and purpose.

We truly are only limited by our imagination and the confidence that we have to let it fly free. Whenever limitations or negativity appear for you just take a moment to stop what you are doing and sing, dance, laugh, or celebrate your way to your next destination. Then, no matter where you end up you will arrive feeling happy and alive.

When I started out on my journey of self-discovery I had no idea what I was getting myself into. Sure, I made a lot of mistakes but I also learned from them and moved on.

I wouldn't be where I am today enjoying a life of freedom and adventure if it wasn't for the decision to get to know more about who I am, what my purpose in being here is, and what hidden treasures of creativity lie waiting in my imagination that could be brought out into the world and enjoyed – this book being one of them

There is a magnificent adventure awaiting all of us, of that I am sure. No matter how young or old we are, whether we are rich or poor, or whether we can't even imagine a better life for ourselves – none of it matters.

What matters is that you get in touch with your most inspired dreams and dare to allow yourself to pursue them without hesitation. The ideas, tools, and techniques in this book will help you do just that if you put aside just five minutes a day to do something different than you usually do so that you can get different results in your life.

Steady growth is bound to happen for you when you do five minutes of practice daily rather than half an hour on some days and none on others. Just like going to the gym and doing reps improves your strength and fitness, doing reps with five-minute meditations or techniques will guarantee that you get results.

As I said at the start: If you are clear in the mind you will be able to find solutions for every problem that arises in your mind. It's only when you can't see a solution that you can feel like you are boxed in with nowhere to go. That's when we start to suffer.

Your first-class, one-way ticket to suffer less and live more is in what you do with the information you have received in this book. From a simple 5-minute mindfulness meditation, to daring to break free from the limiting rules and habits that hold you back in life finding what makes your heart sing, hopefully you found something here that inspires you to be more of who you are.

If you apply just one of the ideas or techniques in this book and put it into practice, it will change your life. I promise. If you want to connect with me there are a few ways to do it. I love to hear how readers take these ideas and apply them to their lives. Whether you have a question that needs answering, or an inspirational story to share, please don't hesitate to write me:

michael@michaelatma.com

Finally, I'd like to invite you to check out even more information, bonus material, and extra resources on the book website. There you will find some additional mind-space exercises that you can download as well as links to some simple mindfulness meditations to help clear your mind and relax your body in just five minutes a day.

www.masteryourmindspace.com

As we reach the end of this book, let this be the beginning of a bigger, brighter, and more enlightened way of living for you and all those you love and cherish.

This moment belongs to you. Today is the day you choose to take control of your life starting with 5-minute exercises to be-here-now and clear your mind. Then, your life will begin to unfold in the most amazing ways. Live fully. Live freely. Be happy.

ABOUT THE AUTHOR

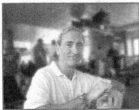

Michael Atma was born and raised in Australia and runs several successful business from his home office. From meditating in different and unusual places every day for the past 17 years, to dedicating his life to helping others to clear their mind, live more fully and follow their dreams. He founded Mindspace Club and wrote *Master Your Mindspace* to teach people who want more control in their life how to have more power, passion, and purpose while awakening their inner brilliance and changing their lives.

He's passionate about meditation, playing the guitar, writing books and songs, and studying the art of Aikido as a physical way to live the principles of creating more mind-space. When he is not developing self-help products, or consulting with clients on how to take control of their personal or business lives, he can usually be found spending time with his three dogs and planning his next ocean-side getaway at some of the most beautiful places in the world.

Meet Michael and receive free mindfulness

and meditation training at:

www.MichaelAtma.com

Your Free Gift

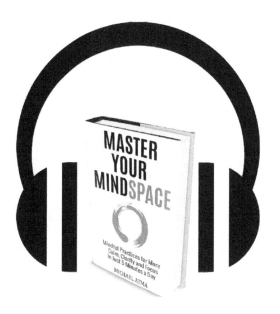

These seven guided meditations will give you greater calm, clarity and focus in just 5-minutes per day.

Or go to:

http://www.masteryourmindspace.com/meditationprogram

Made in the USA
Monee, IL
16 August 2020

38534223R00138